Succeeding in Nursing and Midwifery Educatio

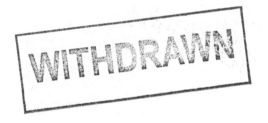

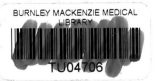

Succeeding in Nursing and Midwifery Education

Edited by

Eddie Meyler
Thames Valley University

and

Steve Trenoweth
Thames Valley University

John Wiley & Sons, Ltd

Other Wiley Editorial Offices

John Wiley & Sons Inc., 111 River Street, Hoboken, NJ 07030, USA

Jossey-Bass, 989 Market Street, San Francisco, CA 94103-1741, USA

Wiley-VCH Verlag GmbH, Boschstr. 12, D-69469 Weinheim, Germany

John Wiley & Sons Australia Ltd, 42 McDougall Street, Milton, Queensland 4064, Australia

John Wiley & Sons (Asia) Pte Ltd, 2 Clementi Loop #02-01, Jin Xing Distripark, Singapore 129809

John Wiley & Sons Canada Ltd, 6045 Freemont Blvd, Mississauga, Ontario, L5R 4J3, Canada

Wiley also publishes its books in a variety of electronic formats. Some content that appears
in print may not be available in electronic books.

Library of Congress Cataloging-in-Publication Data

Succeeding in nursing and midwifery education / edited by Eddie
  Meyler and Steven Trenoweth.
    p. ; cm.
  Includes bibliographical references and index.
  ISBN-13: 978-0-470-03556-6 (pbk. : alk. paper)
  ISBN-10: 0-470-03556-0 (pbk. : alk. paper)
  1. Nursing – Study and teaching. 2. Midwifery – Study and teaching.
I. Meyler, Eddie. II. Trenoweth, Steven.
  [DNLM: 1. Education, Nursing. 2. Midwifery – education.
WY 18 S942 2007]
RT71.S79 2007
610.73076 – dc22

                                            2006026717

British Library Cataloguing in Publication Data

A catalogue record for this book is available from the British Library

ISBN 978-0-470-03556-6 (PB)

Typeset in 10/14 Myriad by Laserwords Private Limited, Chennai, India
Printed and bound in Great Britain by Antony Rowe Ltd, Chippenham, Wiltshire
This book is printed on acid-free paper responsibly manufactured from sustainable forestry
in which at least two trees are planted for each one used for paper production.

Contents

Foreword

by Professor Sandra Jowett

A major challenge for all of us working in education is how best to support our students to enable them to reach their professional and personal potential. It is the responsibility we take most seriously and the source of much of our job satisfaction. Our students join us at very different stages of life and they come with a wide range of attributes and expectations. Some are continuing an unbroken period of full-time education; others have been outside the formal education system for some time and may be returning after a lengthy period of employment or parenting. What they have in common is that they have come to us to develop or enhance their skills and most are seeking qualifications that will enable them to progress professionally. For the particular groups of students for whom this book is written there is a very clear vocational goal, as they have already chosen to study in order to qualify as a nurse or midwife.

I was delighted to hear that my colleagues were compiling this book. Much effort is expended in all universities delivering health and social care programmes to inform and advise prospective students, to develop the study skills of those on programmes and to encourage them to optimize their learning in both academic and work-based settings. What this book does so effectively is to pull together in an accessible and lively format a wealth of experience of providing this input. It covers a wide range of the important issues identified by my colleagues. They know, from years of experience, what anxieties students may have, what practical advice they may value and what support they need in order to benefit from what higher education can provide. The authors have written up this collective wisdom to produce a very upbeat and insightful 'how to' guide.

I learnt a good deal about the aspirations and experiences of pre-registration students when I undertook an evaluation of the implementation of Project 2000 for the Department of Health between 1989 and 1994. Project 2000 changed significantly the way in which courses were delivered, notably by moving such provision into higher education. The findings from the evaluation highlighted the need to address effectively the very varied

educational backgrounds and life experiences of the students, the vital importance c
robust personal support system and the considerable progress that has been made
identifying students' learning needs and providing for them. Others have also comment
on the complexity of the demands placed upon pre-registration students, suggesting t
a proactive and multifaceted approach to student support is required.

This book is a fitting record of my colleagues' contribution to providing this type of suppc
It should be of value to all those thinking of undertaking a nursing or midwifery cou
as well as to those already registered on such programmes. Parents and partners of b
groups are likely to benefit from dipping into it too, because it makes clear the very r
challenges, as well as the joys, of being on these courses. It may help those readers
understand what the student they know is experiencing and perhaps make providing t
all important support a little easier! I trust that, whatever your reason for reading this bo
you will enjoy it and will find it informative and authoritative. It is definitely one to have
the shelf to return to as different issues arise. Here are the voices of some well-inform
'critical friends' who can help with dilemmas and point readers in the right directio
commend this book to you and wish all student readers well on the tough but infinit
rewarding path they have chosen.

Chapter 1

Succeeding in Nursing and Midwifery Education: An Overview

by Eddie Meyler and Steve Trenoweth

We hope you find this book a helpful guide to navigate your journey from thinking abc applying for a programme in nursing or midwifery to qualifying as a healthcare practition The book is not intended as a manual or instruction book, but as a companion to enal you to be successful at the university of your choice, and to get the most out of yc nursing and midwifery programme. Although the book is primarily intended for studer the content of the chapters can be used by academics in supporting students to get t best out on their programme. The sequencing of the chapters is intended to accurat mirror your journey and reflect on the potential challenges and opportunities ahead.

The chapters are written in a conversational style. The authors of each chapter aim to spe to you directly, offering you advice and guidance from their experience in and of nursi and midwifery education. The chapters do not have to be read in sequence although y may choose to do this, but you may also use the book as a resource and dip into t various chapters as the need arises. Each chapter has clear aims and contains useful t and suggestions

An Annotated Overview of the Chapters

The first section is focused on some of the issues you might like to consider in planni to apply for a nursing or midwifery programme. Chapter 2 is written by a student a here you will be able you read first hand an honest view of Sue McGowan's experience a nursing/midwifery programme. She is giving you the sort of advice and guidance s would like to have had!

Chapter 3, How Your Programme is Structured, considers the requirements of nursing a midwifery programmes, in terms of their theory and practice components. In Chapter Applying for a Nursing/Midwifery Programme, you are offered clear guidance on how complete the application process.

Chapter 5, The Student with a Disability, Chronic Health or Learning Needs, deals w important and sensitive issues.. This chapter defines what disability is and provides detail information about the rights and responsibilities of disabled nursing and midwif students. The chapter stresses the importance of disabled students being appreciated a supported by the university so that everyone, regardless of need, has a fair chance succeed.

Chapter 6 is The Interview. In this chapter, the authors' intention is to help you get the best out of the interview to ensure that you secure a place on the programme you wish and at your chosen university. The interview is often a very daunting and anxiety provoking experience and this chapter aims to help you to manage such anxieties. Advice is given about how to create a good impression and how to deal with typical questions that arise at the interview.

The second section is focused on helping you to develop your academic and study skills. Chapter 7 takes a light-hearted look at Using Information Technology and is of particular relevance to you if you have little or no previous experience of using computers. This chapter will help you to get the best out of technology, including some good ideas about purchasing equipment, and how to avoid common disasters that beset students. Chapter 8 is Getting the Most from Your Library. You are advised on how to access a range of support services and specialist library staff who will support you in accessing useful literature for your academic work.

Chapter 9, Becoming Analytical, is designed to help you to write academic essays. This chapter will also help you to become aware of how you can develop in-depth approaches to learning and understanding (in the classroom and in the practice environment) and, importantly, what to do in the face of adversity. The author of this chapter suggests that as you gain experience, both in the classroom and in practice environments, it will become clear that there is no single best or correct way of doing things, and that different people will approach the same issue in a range of different ways.

In Chapter 10, Critiquing the Healthcare Literature, you will gain an insight into the skills of criticism and appreciate why taking a balanced and reasoned view of the literature is an important issue. You will also be introduced to the skills of how to manage, simplify and collate healthcare literature.

In Chapter 11, Organizing and Planning Your Theoretical Assessments, you will be offered an opportunity to think about how to adopt a structured approach to the production of your academic essays. In Chapter 12, How to Write in an Academic Way, you are given advice about the form and style of writing required at universities, while Chapter 13 illustrates How to Reference Your Work and Avoid Plagiarism. In Chapter 14, Making the Most of Assessment Feedback, you will consider how reflection on your theoretical and practice assessments will contribute to your personal and professional development.

The third section is focused on clinical skills development. Chapter 15, Maximizing Yo
Learning in Practice Placements, explains that the practice component of nursing a
midwifery programmes contributes 50% of the programme and therefore it is importa
that you make the most of this experience. This chapter guides you on the preparation y
should undertake to maximise clinical learning opportunities. It is important to be able
identify and respond to your own clinical learning in order to develop new skills that w
equip you for your future professional life.

This theme is developed further in Chapter 16, Developing Your Clinical Skills, where advi
and hints will be contextualized within a clinical skills centre. This is particularly importa
as it is crucial for all healthcare practitioners to be competent in basic life support skil
infection control, safe moving and handling practice and a range of care interventi
skills. An understanding of the concept of 'duty of care' will be nurtured along with t
importance of being able to apply evidence-based findings to clinical practice.

The fourth section is focused on helping you to cope with some of the stresses and strai
that might arise from the programme. In Chapter 17, Surviving the Clinical Environmer
you are offered some advice on how to meet some of the personal challenges that ca
arise. Chapter 18, How to Survive Exams, discusses different types of seen and unsee
assessments and how to deal with examination stress in a positive way. Here, you a
offered guidance on how to plan and manage your revision, reflecting your own person
learning styles.

Chapters 19 and 20 offer advice on obtaining support from your students' union ar
personal tutor respectively. Your personal tutor is an important figure in your educatio
and this chapter offers advice on how to get to know your personal tutor, what suppo
you can expect from him or her and how you might go about developing a productiv
working relationship with them.

Similarly, it is important for you to understand how your students' union can support yo
in your road to success in nursing and midwifery education.

In the final section, we consider issues relating to your development and growth both a
a person and as a practitioner. Initially, we discuss a subject that is not often addressed
nursing and midwifery education. The programme might affect you personally in a numbe
of ways and a degree of personal change through a nursing and midwifery programm
is to be expected. Such changes can be very positive, but may also require you to mak
some adjustments to your personal life. Chapter 21 considers personal change and will k

a vehicle for you to reflect on the impact of change on your professional and personal life. The chapter considers both the positive aspects of change (such as developing your self-confidence and becoming more assertive) and also the challenging side of change and the impact this might have for those closest to you. The chapter helps you to appreciate the importance of being proactive in managing the change process.

In Chapter 22, Preparing Yourself for Your Nursing/Midwifery Career, attention is turned to securing the post that you really want.. A number of searching questions are posed, such as what is the right post for you; how you might support yourself in the transition from student to qualified nurse/midwife; and how to maintain your professional portfolio and develop your career. Chapter 23 gives some final thoughts and offers some suggestions on how to develop you nursing/ midwifery career and how to keep a momentum to your studies.

We hope that you find this book informative and that you will find much in these pages to help you to succeed in your chosen programme.

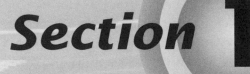

Section 1

Preparing for Nursing and Midwifery Education

In this section, the authors help you to secure a place at the university, and on the programme, of your choice.

Nursing and midwifery programmes can be intellectually stimulating, emotionally challenging, and both life changing and life affirming. It is very important that before you embark upon such education that you are clear as to the nature and structure of the

programme you have chosen, and also that you understand the personal demands t
might place upon you. Among the issues for your consideration are the potential financ
implications of studying full time on the programme, and the possible disruption to yc
family or personal life. Furthermore, if you have a disability, chronic health or learni
needs, you will need to satisfy yourself that you will receive the necessary support to whi
you are entitled.

Once you are clear that you can offer a commitment to your chosen programme, adv
is given on how to ensure a successful application, and how to deal with the stresses a
challenges of the selection interview!

Chapter 2

A Student's Journey

by Sue McGowan

I do not set myself up as an expert on such matters, all I can offer is some thoughts on subject and scraps of advice picked up along the way.

I am writing this mostly from the perspective of a mature student. This is the o perspective I know.

If you are reading this you may be metaphorically standing beside the swimming p of nurse/midwifery education wondering whether to dive in, dip a toe or just sit in a lounger and watch the others. Presumably you know a little about what the program and what nursing or midwifery involves. You will know that it bears little resemblar to the popular television dramas – dashing to save a patient's life one minute and th getting up to mischief with a doctor among the bedpans the next minute.

You may be a school leaver or, like myself, a mature person for whom school and colle are a dim and distant memory. Both groups have their positive and negative aspects. T school leavers will know what a book looks like, will know how to use a computer and have been used to studying. However, you may be fed up with learning and not totally s of what you want from life. The more mature among you may have had some experier of caring, either for your children or for elderly relatives. You are more likely to be settle your personal life and know 'who you are'. Having said this it may be a long time since y last studied and it can be a daunting prospect. The closest I had got to academic writ in the last 21 years was compiling the weekly grocery list. Add to this reading and critic analysing the television guide and you will understand my level.

You may be looking at a prospectus and become daunted at the prospect of studying n subjects. For instance, you may have hated science at school and in turn you were not v good at it. Do not let this put you off. At school science was an alien concept to me. C look at a Bunsen burner and I would feel faint. During my nursing programme I found enjoyment and understanding of the subject, which took me totally by surprise. This v because it had relevance to my future career.

Nursing and midwifery programmes vary greatly depending on the institution providi the programmes. All comprise periods of university-based theory alternated with ti spent in the field on clinical placements. Placements can be everything you ever dream of or your worst nightmare depending on the setting, the staff and your perceptions. C of the things that this programme has taught me is that nurses are human beings t strange as it may seem. There are nice nurses and there are not so nice nurses. There some who will be incredibly supportive and an inspiration and there will be others who will inspire you to think some very uncharitable thoughts while you are with them.

Placements are a necessary delight/evil and have to be enjoyed/endured. As long as you remain polite but assertive, helpful and eager to learn you will emerge relatively unscathed. When on placement remember to ask questions. Not all healthcare professionals will be approachable and of course can be very busy and may not welcome intrusion from students. However, choose your moments and you will encounter those who relish passing on their wisdom. Take advantage of these people, in the academic sense of course. Be interested in what they have to say, not only will it boost your knowledge but also it is flattering and we all like a bit of flattery.

One of the most important tips I can give you is to purchase and get to know how to use a computer or 'PC', as I believe it is known. Slightly older students may think that a PC is a gentleman who carries a truncheon and that a floppy disk relates to back trouble. Becoming computer literate is a necessity. You will be able to produce beautifully typed assignments, even if you only use two fingers, and the Internet is essential for looking up facts and figures and journal articles. At assignment time you will need to do a lot of research and, unless you want to live in the university library, having a computer at your disposal is a must.

If you have just left school you will find the bursary useful, as it may be the first time you have earned a monthly salary. Older students might find it a struggle. You may be leaving paid employment to undertake the programme and the financial side needs careful consideration. Many students join a 'nurse bank' to work shifts and also gain extra hands-on experience. If you do work extra shifts, be sensible and do not over-burden yourself. You will need time to study and trying to cram everything in will only result in more stress. Financial planning is needed before embarking on a programme to avoid hardship later on. As your programme progresses you will need to be very focused and money worries can be very distracting.

School leavers may see their friends go off to university to study other subjects, which require, how shall I put it, less commitment. They will get drunk, wake up hugging a traffic cone and chuck in a bit of studying for good measure. You will not be able to enter into such debauchery. On the first day we were reminded that as student nurses we were expected to act in a manner befitting our status. In other words, not to bring the name of nurses into disrepute.

I cannot stress too heavily how important it is to plan and get organized! Before you st
your programme it is useful to do a little background reading. Whatever branch of nursi
you are studying you will be learning about anatomy, physiology, psychology and aspe
of sociology. Getting a basic grasp of these before you enter the classroom makes for few
surprises later on.

Planning and preparing well beforehand means you need not turn into a raging, obnoxio
beast around the time that your assignment is due in. If you want to have any friends
family left when you have finished the programme then you need to let them know th
at certain times you will not be able to perform your usual 'social functions'. This can al
be useful when trying to avoid housework. Having said that, it is amazing how attractive
week's worth of laundry becomes when you should be working on your essay.

There are lots of study guides published that tell you to reserve a place in the home whe
you can work uninterrupted and keep all your materials in one place. This is useful b
not possible for everyone. At the very least have a large box where you can keep fil
of notes, reports and articles. Get into the habit of never throwing anything away. A
newspaper or journal article may come in useful one day and you can find useful b
of information in the unlikeliest of publications. Don't buy loads of books before yo
programme starts. Your university will provide you with a list of suggested titles. Boo
are very expensive. You could ask any ex-students if they have any to sell or look on t
Internet for secondhand books. A well-written anatomy and physiology book will be vital
the first year. Helpful, too, is the fact that human anatomy, unlike nursing/midwifery theo
and procedures, does not change. Well, hopefully it doesn't unless of course there is
unexpected discovery of a new organ. As students, we are encouraged to use up-to-da
information, such as journal articles, which can be found in libraries or on the Intern
I have bought books I have hardly used because they were out of date as soon as th
appeared on the shelves. They are, however, very useful for propping up wonky coff
tables.

Have you seen a puppy as it first opens its eyes? It blinks at the light and peers out into th
alien world not really knowing what is going on. This is how you may feel when startir
at university, although *you* may already be house trained. When you get used to yo
lecturers and having to study you will feel that you have been a student all your life. If yo
are older you will find that there are a lot of mature students out there so you won't b

lonely. If you are young, well there are younger people there too so you will not feel you have been transported to an old folks' home.

Along with my fellow students I have been told countless times to make the most of being a student. To ask questions and not to be afraid of trying things and failing. It has taken me until now to realize that it is only by questions and answers that lecturers know you are following what is going on. It can be difficult for the more timid of us to speak up in class. However, we are all adults and no one will laugh at you if you give the 'wrong' answer – but think of the thrill when you get one right! Now I am in my third year and as the prospect of being let loose on the poor unsuspecting patients draws near I wish I had relished my student status more.

Nursing or midwifery is not glamorous and you will need a strong stomach. You will encounter bodily fluids that you never knew existed. It is, however, one of the most rewarding careers you can have. One where even the seemingly simplest actions such as holding someone's hand and being there for them when they are distressed can make a world of difference. When a person is ill and in hospital they are at their most vulnerable. If they trust you enough to turn to you for support, it is a great privilege and a huge responsibility.

There are many avenues open to qualified nurses and midwives, and these will expand in the future. For example, nurses and midwives are taking over roles that were once the sole domain of doctors, such as prescribing medication. You can work on a ward, in the community and in clinics. You can specialize, work overseas or teach.

I will not bother to tell you that nursing and midwifery is not just a job but a vocation. You will probably have heard it all before and, although I think it is true, it has been used as a tactic by various governments in order to keep nurses' pay to a minimum, so I will leave it well alone. Suffice to say that our love for our work does not help to pay the mortgage! Anyway, the pay is improving!

I hope my befuddled rantings have not put you off. Nurse and midwifery training can be an enriching experience. Whatever your age you will discover qualities you didn't know you had. You will learn new skills, meet new people and at the end of it be qualified in one of the most important and rewarding careers. So there you are beside the swimming pool of nursing or midwifery education. Get out of that sun lounger and jump in!

Tips

- Don't become daunted by the prospect of study
- Ask questions!
- Don't be afraid of speaking up
- Plan before and during the nursing/midwifery programme
- Don't buy too many books before the programme starts
- Make the most of being a student!

Chapter 3

How Your Programme is Structured

by Eddie Meyler and David Stroud

This chapter considers:

- **The structure of nursing and midwifery programmes**
- **The regulatory framework of nursing and midwifery programmes**
- **Statutory requirements to register as a nurse or midwife**
- **What you will study on your programme**
- **The importance of self directed study.**

Although nursing and midwifery programmes must follow approved templates l down by the Nursing and Midwifery Council (NMC) (NMC 2004a; NMC 2004b), there differences in the way programmes are delivered. Universities are responding to chang in the demographics of the nursing and midwifery student population by trying to prov a flexible, more family-friendly timetable. Nevertheless, nursing and midwifery care m be provided on a 24-hour, 7-day week basis and students must experience all aspects care. So be prepared for this!

Introduction

Nursing and midwifery education is structured to meet both the academic demands of university and the professional expectations of the NMC. The NMC establishes standa and requirements for programmes leading to professional registration. Furthermo healthcare providers, such as the National Health Service (NHS), have expectations t nursing and midwifery education will make you a competent and reliable employee w will be able to deliver safe and effective care.

You should be aware that the structure of your programme differs from traditio university programmes and that these may place additional demands on you and y time. You will have to cope with the demands of both the university and health-c environments, while frequently adjusting to a range of different health and social c teams. There is also travel to, and from, clinical placements to take into account. Y programme will be structured around university term times that will not necessa coincide with your children's school holidays. Furthermore, the teaching day and we are varied and reflect different patterns from one university to another, which might h implications for childcare responsibilities. These are important issues that you will nee consider and adjust to and you might need to make appropriate personal arrangeme before commencing your programme of study.

Structure of the Midwifery Programme

The NMC (2004a) stipulates that the length of the pre-registration midwifery program should not be less than three years, equivalent to 156 weeks' full-time (where each y contains 45 programmed weeks). When delivered full time the student should compl in five years, including interruptions, and seven years if part-time. Where the studen already registered with the NMC as an Adult Nurse (Level 1), the length of the program should not be less than 18 months, equivalent to 78 weeks' full time, or equivalent pro rata for part-time programmes.

The emphasis in midwifery programmes is on providing care for, and promoting the health of, women and babies. In addition, clinical placements should provide experience of different methods of midwifery care, such as home births, midwife-led units and birth centres. The balance between theory and practice is similar to that of nursing, 50% clinical practice and 50% theory.

The Midwifery programme pre-registration proficiencies (NMC 2004a) also encompass four domains:

- Effective Midwifery Practice (e.g. communicate effectively with women and their families throughout the pre-conception, antenatal, intrapartum and postnatal periods)
- Professional and Ethical Practice (e.g. you will need to practise in accordance with the NMC Code of Professional Conduct; identify unsafe practice and respond appropriately to ensure safe outcomes, etc.)
- Developing the Individual Midwife and Others (e.g. demonstrate effective working across professional boundaries and develop professional networks)
- Achieving Quality Care Through Evaluation and Research (e.g. by applying relevant knowledge to the midwife's own practice and disseminating critically appraised good practice).

Structure of the Nursing Programme

The NMC (2004b) states that the nursing programme must consist of at least 4600 hours spread over three years and divided equally between theory and practice. In order to register with the NMC, you will need to complete *all* theory and practice hours. Excellent attendance, therefore, both at university and in the practice component of the programme is essential and your attendance will be closely monitored. Some universities have part-time arrangements, often structured around school terms for the convenience of students who have children. Although some students take breaks for personal or family reasons, all nursing programmes must usually be completed within five years from the starting date, including interruptions. This extends to seven years on part-time programmes.

The first year of the nursing programme is called the Common Foundation Programme (often referred to simply as the CFP). The CFP will introduce you to principles and practice

of care in a range of health and social care settings. Upon successful completion
the foundation year you will go on to the second part of the programme – the Bran
programme where you will develop further the knowledge and skills to work within yo
chosen specialist area – adult, mental health, child and learning disability nursing.

You need to bear in mind that the CFP normally has to be successfully completed before yo
can progress to any of the branches of nursing. However, from 1 September 2006 you ha
up to an additional 12 weeks to complete the foundation year from the commencem
of the second year of the programme (NMC Circular 16/2006).

The Nursing programme pre-registration proficiencies (NMC 2004b) are encompass
within four domains:

- Professional and Ethical Practice (e.g. you will need to practise in accordance with
  NMC Code of Professional Conduct; identify unsafe practice and respond appropriat
  to ensure safe outcomes, etc.)
- Care Delivery (e.g. you will need to utilize a range of effective communication a
  engagement skills; consult with patients, clients and groups to identify their need a
  desire for health promotion advice)
- Care Management (e.g. use appropriate risk assessment tools to identify actual a
  potential risks; establish and maintain collaborative working relationships with hea
  and social care teams and others)
- Personal and Professional Development (e.g. identify one's own personal and professio
  development needs by engaging in activities such as reflection).

Taking a Break

Your programme is designed to accommodate some degree of flexibility should yo
need to take a break. For example, there is some provision made for maternity lea
The Department of Health allows students to receive up to 45 weeks of bursary p
ments while on maternity leave. However, this is not the same as an employm
right, because taking time off to have a baby will naturally interfere with your abi
to meet the standard regulatory requirements of your programme. That is, follow
maternity leave you will need to rejoin the programme at an appropriate point in or
to make up the time that you have missed from the programme. The financial arran
ments for students intending to take time out from their programme and other iss

related to bursary payment can be obtained on the NHS Student Grants Unit website www.nhsstudentgrants.co.uk.

If you need to take time off from the programme for any reason, the start and end dates of this absence need to be discussed and agreed between you and your personal tutor or programme leader.

The Programme in More Detail

Teaching methods

The way the university teaches might be different from what you have experienced previously. The university model values individual learning and students' contributions in tutorials and seminars. You will also be given personal tutorial support and guidance, although the way this is done varies from one university to another.

Teaching will include lectures, small group tutorials, discussion groups and some universities will even make use of simulations of care situations in clinical skills centres, or skills laboratories using sophisticated electronic mannequins or even real life actors! It might also make use of traditional laboratories so that you may undertake specific physiological or biochemical experiments. Increasingly, universities are making use of electronic resources that you will be encouraged to use to support and further develop your knowledge and understanding of particular healthcare issues. While it is recognized that we all have our preferred learning style, you will still need to adapt to the university's methods and patterns of teaching.

You might hear frequent reference to you, as a student, being an 'adult' learner. This means that you are expected to be actively involved in, and take personal responsibility for, your learning. There is likely to be an emphasis placed on learning with, and from, other students, by undertaking group projects. You might also facilitate presentations on a variety of topics and healthcare issues to fellow students and lecturers. This will not only help you to develop a knowledge base, but will also help you to develop your confidence in speaking in front of a group.

Levels of study

Nursing programmes are run at diploma and degree level. In general, the differences between these academic levels are indicated by two important considerations: the

autonomy of the learner (i.e. the degree to which the learner is self-directed) and *respons*
ity (i.e. the degree to which students become personally responsible for their own learni
(SEEC 2002). Often degree students are expected to have a greater range, and depth
detail, in their academic knowledge. For example, the degree level student will be expec
to analyse data with relatively little guidance using a comprehensive range of literatur
order to identify and offer novel solutions to complex clinical problems. A diploma stud
however, might be expected to have a detailed knowledge of important and relev
research and literature, and would be able to compare and contrast competing theo
and ideas in order to choose appropriate methods for the resolution of clinical problem

There are obviously more academic demands placed upon degree students, wh
undoubtedly will require a higher level of personal commitment and time required
complete theoretical assessments.

Modules of study

A module is a defined unit of study built around particular themes. Nursing and midwif
modules of study are credit rated. The most common structure is for a single module
have 20 credits and a double module to have 40 credits. In order to achieve a diplo
you will usually need to undertake sufficient modules to obtain 240 academic credit
diploma level, whereas to obtain a degree you will require 360 credits at degree le
However, please be aware that universities will have different regulations in relation
the amount of credits required to obtain these qualifications. If you are undertaking
honours degree, you are likely to be required to undertake a dissertation – an extend
assignment where, for example, you will undertake an in-depth and detailed literat
review and analysis on a chosen subject.

What You Need to Study

The programmes are designed for you to achieve a broad range of physical and psyc
logical care skills. Midwifery and each of the branches of nursing will cover all the follow
topics, although the emphasis placed upon each will differ depending on your cho
field of study.

Care skills

Nursing and midwifery care encompasses the technical knowledge and skills, perso
attitudes and values that are required to provide help and assistance to people with he
needs.

Some of these care skills are very obvious. For example, most people are used to seeing nurses and midwives using their skills in TV hospital soaps. These are entertaining works of fiction which use dramatic events to tell a story. While nursing and midwifery care can involve delivering babies, defibrillating patients, cleaning and dressing wounds, setting up intravenous lines, and so on, the reality can be less dramatic! The focus can be on 'hidden' care skills, that is, aspects of care which are more subtle and not so obvious, an important precursor of which is the ability to feel concern, and empathize with your patients. Comforting an anxious pre-operative patient is an important aspect of care. It is not dramatic. It is very subtle and of enormous potential value to the psychological health of the patient.

Record keeping

A very important skill to learn is that of effective record keeping. In fact, the NMC states that this is a reflection of the quality of the care you provide (NMC 2005). The importance of nurses and midwives being able to maintain accurate records cannot be overstated and the programme will emphasize the legal aspects of keeping accurate health-related records.

Anything written by a nurse or midwife becomes a legal document. Badly kept records can lead to mistakes, the consequences of which can be serious, sometimes leading to legal or disciplinary action. Good record keeping not only facilitates effective nursing care, but also helps staff reflect and learn, enhances clinical supervision and can be used in research. In fact, the NMC feels that the quality of nursing records is a reflection of the standards of care that are provided. Report writing is a skill to be learnt – it is not, as some people think, as easy as writing a personal diary or writing a letter to a friend. Reading quality journal articles or textbooks is a good way to help you gain an appreciation of more formal writing styles.

Medication management

The administration of medication is an important aspect of nursing and midwifery practice (NMC 2004c). In addition to developing your knowledge about the types of medicine, maximum and therapeutic ranges of dosages, effects and side effects, you will need to become skilled in its safe administration. You will need to learn about the many routes in the administration of medication (e.g. oral, topical, rectal, subcutaneous, intramuscular, intravenous, etc.). Additionally, there are ethical issues in respect of medication management that you must be mindful of. For example, it is essential to ensure that the patient has full information regarding their medication and has given their meaningful and informed consent.

Please remember that the NMC requires that students are always supervised in administration of medication.

Science

It is very important that you develop your knowledge in the sciences, such as anato physiology, biology, chemistry, biochemistry and pharmacology. This knowledge enable you to appreciate the effect of disease processes on the body. It is important, example, to fully understand the effects of the body's systems (e.g. circulatory, cen nervous and immune systems) on health and illness. A common concern in recent yea that nurses do not have enough knowledge of these sciences.

Social sciences

Social science is the study of human behaviour and society and this knowledge is import as health care exists within a social and political context. For example, access to he might depend upon issues such as one's social background and education. These important sociological, and possibly political, ideas that you will need to explore du the programme. Additionally, you will learn how family and cultural issues affect peop health, including the effect of unemployment, housing and social class. You will also le how ethnicity and gender are important issues to consider as factors that influence acc to, and expectations of, health care.

Similarly, in psychology, you will learn about how people's experiences, their thoug beliefs and attitudes can affect how they perceive themselves and that this, in turn, mi affect their recovery. You will learn about group behaviour, including how people themselves and others, and how they act and react to each other and to life in general

Developing communication skills and effective team working

You will learn the importance of and how to develop therapeutic relationships with pati and their families. It is therefore very important that you have a good understanc of self-presentation and that you are able to utilize effective verbal and non-ve communication skills. Furthermore, as a nurse or midwife you will need to communic with a wide range of colleagues and agencies, including other nurses, general practitior specialist consultants, social workers, volunteers, radiographers and pharmacists. Moc health care is built on teamwork.

Nurses have to learn to meet the challenges of life and death. Therefore, the programme will enable you to deal with the emotional effects of bad news, and how to communicate this to individuals and families. It is important to remember, though, that patients do recover or adapt to changes in their health status and express gratitude to nurses/midwives who have helped them.

Understanding personal reactions to ill health

Health is more complex than many people realize, often meaning different things to different people. Nurses and midwives need to understand the nature of health and illness, and how this might be influenced by one's culture and personal experience.

As a student, you will need to understand how people of all ages respond to illness. Reactions to a diagnosis of a serious illness, such as cancer, vary from cycling around the world to raise money for charity to withdrawing from life and waiting to die. The nurse/midwife has to learn to understand, respond to, and accept, the diverse range of their client's physical, social and psychological responses to illness.

Practising ethically

The programme should trigger ethical and legal questions for you. It is important for you to participate in learning events, such as debates, as these will help you not only to clarify ethical arguments on both sides of an issue, but will assist you to develop skills of public speaking and assertion.

For example, where do you stand in these issues?

- Do you believe that overweight people should take more responsibility for their own health?
- Do you believe that teenagers should take more precautions not to get pregnant?
- Do you feel that people with mental illness are dangerous?
- Do you believe that smokers should be denied life saving surgery? If you believe this to be the case, how would you rationalize this in terms of your duty of care?

Understanding our own sense of personal morality (i.e. your own sense of what is right and wrong) and how we respond ethically is part of nursing and is an essential precursor to engaging in effective ethical practice. The programme will challenge some of your existing beliefs and ask you to consider how you might provide care to those who have different personal moral frameworks from yourself.

Health promotion

Modern nursing and midwifery programmes emphasize the importance of promot
health and the prevention of illness. You will learn to empower people to take responsibi
for their own health in the areas of diet, safe sex, exercise and healthy living, and adv
them about screening for hidden diseases such as breast or prostate cancer and high blc
pressure.

Key skills

Nursing and midwifery programmes stress the importance of attaining a wide range
'key skills' as a complement to the specialist knowledge and skills required to deli
health care. Therefore, nursing and midwifery programmes will assist you in y
development of such skills, for example the ability to work with numbers, commu
cation, improving one's own learning and performance, information and communicat
technology, problem solving and working with others. You may also be offered
opportunity to take additional qualifications within your programme to demonstrate y
attainment of certain key skills. For example, some universities offer the opportunity
undertake the European Computer Driving Licence (ECDL) (for further information
`www.ecdl.com/publisher/index.jsp`).

Management

Management is an essential subject for nurses and midwives. This involves all types
management – of patient care, resources, personnel, stress, time, and yourself. Working
part of a team, you need to know how to get the best out of yourself and your colleagu
Therefore management, leadership and teamwork will be themes in your programme
required by the NMC (NMC 2004a; NMC 2004b). As a practitioner of the future, you ne
to be able to lead a multiprofessional team and advocate for your patients in a variety
health and social care settings.

Evidence-based practice

At this stage you might feel overwhelmed by the volume and complexity of knowlec
and ideas you will have to absorb. But take heart, you will also be taught how
learn and how to search for the information you need. Evidence-based practice will
a major part of your studies in both nursing and midwifery. This includes doing
word searches in databases in order to ascertain which nursing and midwifery care a

interventions are known to be effective. These skills are discussed in more detail in Section 2 of this book.

In the past, health care was based on tradition and habit. For instance, patients were always fasted from midnight before an operation; it was assumed that bed rest was necessary for recovery; that hospital was the place to be when you were ill; and that babies should be born in maternity units. All these ideas have been challenged in recent years. Ideas and values about health and illness have changed and continue to evolve, and you will have a key role in determining how patients will be cared for in the future. Nursing and midwifery education will encourage and develop your reflective and analytical skills and to consider new, improved ways of providing care. The important thing to remember is that modern healthcare practice should be based on sound research evidence. That is, our practice must be based on the interventions that will lead to improved clinical outcomes for our patients.

Clinical learning

On the practice part of your programme you will become aware of how nursing/midwifery theory underpins practice. You will learn the interpersonal skills involved in dealing with patients, their relatives and other staff, and the relationship between physical and psychological health. The ultimate aim is to be able to deliver effective, safe nursing/midwifery care.

You will have the opportunity to learn how to provide care for patients and their families in a variety of settings, both in the hospital and community, and in the voluntary and private sector. More treatment is now being carried out in general practitioner surgeries.

Interprofessional clinical learning is an increasingly common and important part of modern health care which, it is hoped, will lead to better teamwork and improved patient care. This means that all disciplines, such as nurses, midwives, doctors, social workers and occupational therapists, learn and deliver care together rather than separately. Therefore you may find yourself attending lectures with people other than nurses or midwives. A multidisciplinary approach will certainly be the norm in ward rounds and case conferences on clinical placements.

Being Self-Directed

Your nursing and midwifery programme is structured around the essential skills, knowledge and attitudes you need to develop to practise safely and competently in modern healthcare

environments. In this chapter, we have emphasized the formal structured content th
your university will provide for you. However, as an adult learner you will also be expect
to develop and pursue your own personal interests in healthcare related topics, or issu
that have arisen from your module or programme. You will need to develop your o
structure to make full use of any self-directed study time that is allocated.

Tips

- Find out as much as you can about nursing and midwifery education before applying
  a programme
- Use the Internet to find information about individual universities and how their spec
  programme is organized
- If you choose nursing, decide which branch interests you most
- Be realistic about level of study – would a degree or a diploma programme be better
  you?

References and Further Reading

NMC (2004a) *Standards of Proficiency for Pre-Registration Midwifery Education.* Lond
NMC. Available at: `www.nmc-uk.org/aFrameDisplay.aspx?Docume`
`ID=171`

NMC (2004b) *Standards of Proficiency for Pre-Registration Nursing Education.* London, NM
Available at: `www.nmc-uk.org/aFrameDisplay.aspx?DocumentID=328`

NMC (2004c) *Guidelines for Administration of Medicines.* London, NMC. Available
`www.nmc-uk.org/aFrameDisplay.aspx?DocumentID=221`

NMC (2005) *Guidelines for Records and Record Keeping.* London, NMC. Available
`www.nmc-uk.org/aFrameDisplay.aspx?DocumentID=1120`

SEEC (2002) *SEEC Level Credit Descriptors 2001.* Available at: `www.seec-office.org.u`
`creditleveldescriptors2001.pdf`

World Health Organization (WHO) (2006) *Constitution of the World Health Organizati*
Available at: `www.searo.who.int/LinkFiles/About_SEARO_const.pdf`

Chapter 4

Applying for a Nursing/Midwifery Programme

by Denise Burley

This chapter considers:

- **Issues that you might like to consider before making an application**

- **How to choose the university that is right for you**

- **Making an application to join a nursing or midwifery programme via Universities and Colleges Admissions Service (UCAS) or direct to the university**

- **The information required in support of your application.**

Introduction

The traditional profile of a student nurse/midwife has changed in recent years. Previou
the applicants for nursing and midwifery programmes were predominantly white fema
and aged approximately 18 on entry. Many candidates came into a nursing career strai
from school, with either General Certificate of Education (GCE) 'A' levels or Gene
Certificate of Secondary Education (GCSE) (or equivalent) qualifications. While this v
the norm in the past, over the last 10–15 years there has been a major change regard
applicants and the picture now is very different. Although there is a minimum age limi
17 1/2 years for entry, there is no upper age limit and we are increasingly seeing stude
in their 30s and 40s or older entering university. In addition, the myth of nursing a
midwifery being a female profession is slowly being eroded as more men seek to join
profession.

Points to Consider Before Applying

Before you apply, it is worth taking some time out to consider the implications for y
in undertaking the nursing/midwifery programme. For example, I would suggest that y
consider how it might it affect you and possibly your family; what might the finan
implications be? Are there any implications for child care? At what academic level mi
you wish to study? Here, I will focus on some important, preliminary issues that you n
wish to consider.

The right programme

The first and most obvious issue to consider is your choice of programme. Would y
like to become a midwife? Are you interested in nursing? If you want to becom
nurse, what field of nursing attracts you? There are four branches of nursing – ad
mental health, child and learning disability. It is important that you consider and ma
your selection with care. Although it is not unusual for students to want to char
branch once the programme has started, this may not always be possible. If you
unsure, then contact a local hospital or maternity unit and see if you can have
chat to a midwife or nurse about their role. It might even be possible to spend so
time in the clinical area. I would also advise visiting the National Health Service (NI
Careers website – www.nhscareers.nhs.uk/home.html. This has some very use
background information for you to consider.

Financial implications

Students who apply for the nursing, midwifery and operating department practitioner diploma programmes will be eligible for a bursary if they *have been resident in the United Kingdom, Channel Islands or the Isle of Man for three years continuously preceding, and on, the first day of the programme and have settled in the United Kingdom (within the meaning of the Immigration Act 1971).* It is very important to be aware of the amount of bursary you are entitled to as financial worries will affect your ability to study effectively.

Students receive a bursary from the NHS Student Grants Unit (www.nhsstudentgrants .co.uk). This is a standard amount per year with an increased amount if you are based in London. If you have dependants you still receive the standard bursary and this will not affect 'child benefit'. However, other benefits may be affected and therefore it is important to investigate the financial implications here before you commence the programme (see www.dwp.gov.uk/lifeevent/workage for further guidance). Unfortunately, some students do not research this aspect before coming on to the programme and then find that they have to leave their programme because they cannot manage financially when their benefits are reduced or removed. It is also important to discuss this with the NHS Student Grants Unit as it might be possible to receive a means-tested 'dependant's allowance'.

The bursary is paid on a monthly basis and the amount paid will depend upon your age at the start of the programme. There is a different rate for students who are aged under 26 at the start of the programme from those aged over 26 at the beginning of their programme.

You should also be aware that there are different financial arrangements for those who wish to undertake the degree option of the nursing and midwifery programme. In essence, if you elect to undertake the degree pathway then you will move from a 'non-means-tested' bursary to a 'means-tested' bursary. This may have an impact on how much you receive so it is crucial that you investigate this thoroughly before committing yourself to this higher level of study.

If you have been working previously then it is important to be clear regarding the amount of bursary being paid so that you can make plans to cope with the reduction in income. Some students take on additional jobs to supplement their income while at university and receiving a bursary. While part-time working is for many a financial necessity it is important to remember that nursing and midwifery programmes are full time. There is

an expectation that students will need to spend considerable time studying, researchi
topics and reading in depth about nursing and midwifery practice.

While you should usually expect your bursary to be paid at the commencement of t
programme, an important issue here that you will need to consider is that payment
bursaries can be delayed for many reasons. It is advisable that you plan to make suita
financial arrangements in this eventuality.

Child care

In general, childcare facilities, such as crèches, are not provided by universities. If y
have childcare responsibilities, you will need to consider the impact of the programr
in particular, acknowledging that you will be required to work unsocial hours during t
practice part of the programme. This is essential as nurses and midwives provide ca
24-hours a day, 7-days a week.

Academic level

Many universities offer a degree option as part of the programme. Often you will r
need to state your intention to study at this academic level at the commencement
the programme. The precise details of the diploma and degree options can vary betwe
universities.

Finding the Right University

Your application is part of a two way process – the university will want to ensure that y
are the right candidate for them but also you must be sure that the university is right
you too! It is important to consider carefully issues that lead to selecting the university t
best suits your needs.

Doing some homework

It is important to do some homework regarding nurse or midwifery education. Try to fi
out what you can about the university. It is often difficult to know if you want to atten
university until you see the environment for yourself. I would strongly recommend taki
some time to visit the various universities of your choice. This is true of any situati
whether it be a new job or perhaps a school for one of your children. You may, howev

have some prior knowledge of the university. Perhaps a friend, neighbour or relative has already studied there. If you know someone who has had a good experience then you are more likely to think positively about the university. This is true for us all when we think of other situations; recommendations from friends and acquaintances can be a very powerful persuasive force.

Another way to gain information is to go to the university's website. All universities and NHS Trusts have websites that are accessible to the general public. You can also go to the Quality Assurance Agency's website (www.qaa.ac.uk) and read the most recent quality review of healthcare programmes at your chosen university. The Agency's aim is to safeguard the public through maintaining the standard of qualifications and encouraging ongoing improvement in higher education.

Location

Do you want to move away from home or would you prefer to attend a university that is situated near to where you are already living? You may have some constraints such as family or personal commitments that prevent you moving away from the area or from making a wider choice. There are a few issues here that you will need to consider:

- Is the university near to where you live?
- If you have to travel, will you need a car? Is there public transport available to take you to the various hospital and community sites?
- If there is a cost associated with travel, will this be affordable considering you might be on a reduced income during the programme?
- Investigate the location of areas where you will be undertaking the practice part of the programme. As it is common for universities to be in partnership with NHS Trusts and community, voluntary and private services that cover a wide geographical area, travel can be expensive. It is important to remember that if you are working within a hospital in-patient setting that shifts can begin as early as 6.30 a.m.

Making an Application Via UCAS

You may know exactly which university you wish to apply to and may wish to explore if it is possible to make a direct application to them. However, you may wish to look further afield and to consider a number of universities in different areas of the country or different towns and cities. To help you to do this, you might like to visit the University and

Colleges Admissions Service (UCAS) website (www.ucas.com) which also provides use
information such as:

- Background information about a particular university
- Outline of the application system
- Types of programmes
- Academic requirements
- When to apply
- How to apply.

If you have decided to make an application through UCAS rather than directly to c
university then the application form allows you to list several universities, allowing you
state a preference. The advantage of this form of application is that you will only have
complete an application form once. The information is held centrally by UCAS and sent
the university that you nominate as a preference.

This application process will incur a fee. If you wish to consider just one nursing or midwif
programme at a specific university then UCAS will charge less than if you wish to apply
several universities.

Making a Direct Application

The first step in making a direct application is to contact the university recru
ment/admission department. There is usually a telephone helpline to request an applicati
form and prospectus. However, many universities will have the facility to download th
current prospectus and application forms from their website. This is possibly the quicke
most practical and environmentally friendly way to apply! However, do remember to ke
a copy of the completed online application form. Do not feel intimidated and if you ,
not comfortable with completing the form online and submitting it, then send a copy
the usual way, in the post.

While the majority of universities will send out electronic application packs (includi
application forms), you may still be asked to complete a 'hard' or paper copy. When y
receive the application form it is a good idea to photocopy it. It is really important to ta
time to ensure your application is completed accurately, neatly and legibly, and is w
presented as this will help to create a good impression of you. Once you have complet
your application form it is essential that you keep a photocopy before you return it
the university, particularly if you are making several applications as you will find that ea

university will ask very similar questions. Also, of course, if you have a copy of your original application form for each university, then before attending for interview you can look at it to refresh your memory!

The application pack will have details about how to complete the forms, usually asking you to use a black pen. This is a practical point as black pen shows up more clearly when photocopied (and is therefore easier to read) and most application forms have to be photocopied at least once.

Do not send original Birth/Marriage or Educational certificates in the ordinary post (you have no way of tracking the post or recourse if your letter and its contents are lost). If you have been asked to provide an original certificate, which is not unusual, then send them by either Registered Post or Special Delivery. While this is more expensive, it is a lot cheaper and less timeconsuming than having to get replacement documents. In your covering letter with the application form and original certificates you should state that you have used either 'Registered Post/Special Delivery' or an equivalent and ask for the original certificates to be returned to you using the same system. Some universities, however, may ask you to simply bring your original certificates with you to the interview.

If you are writing a covering letter, then try to keep this brief. You should confirm in this letter that you are submitting your application for the programme (name the programme and the month it begins) and also indicate all the enclosures such as certificates (name each one that they should expect to find) that are included. The admissions office/recruitment department (universities have their own specific name for the department dealing with this activity) will then know what to check as well as what you are expecting to be returned and by what postal method. Occasionally, some universities may keep the documentation until you attend for interview and then return it to you in person. However, these are important documents and you may need them if you have other interviews or for other personal reasons that you do not wish or need to disclose. If there is a delay in returning your certificates then it is perfectly reasonable for you to request that they are returned to you before the interview date.

Information Required

Eligibility

You can apply for a nursing or midwifery programme if you are a British or European Economic Area (EEA) national or have indefinite leave to remain within the country.

The university might ask to see evidence to prove that you are legally allowed reside in this country. If you are not an EEA national, you may still apply for a S dent Visa to undertake the nursing or midwifery programme in England. For furth information, consult the Home Office's Immigration and Nationality Directorate webs www.ind.homeoffice.gov.uk.

Qualifications

When you apply for a nursing or midwifery programme, you are asked to list y qualifications, which enables the admissions office of the university to decide whether y have the required entry qualifications. In general, the *minimum* entry requirements are

- 5 GCSE or GCE (O Levels) of at least Grade C (including English) or equivalent (the midwifery programme requires a Science subject and/or Mathematics)
- An approved Access to Higher Education course
- General National Vocational Qualification (GNVQ) Advanced Level or National Vocational Qualification (NVQ) Level 3
- Edexcel/Business & Technology Education Council (BTEC) National or Higher National Diploma.

Please note that there is a slight variation in these minimum entry requirements in Scotla and Northern Ireland and that some universities may ask for more than the above minim qualifications.

If you obtained your qualifications from another country, then these will have to be auth ticated, verified and the standard agreed. This is undertaken for universities by the Natio Recognition Information Centre for the United Kingdom (NARIC) (www.naric.org.u NARIC is the organization that compares UK qualifications with those around the world a advises as to the standing of the overseas qualifications and whether they are at the le expected for entry to the nursing and midwifery programme that you have applied for

Once this comparison has been undertaken, you may be advised to take further course order to be eligible for the programme of your choice.

Further/supporting information

On most application forms there is a question asking you to give reasons why you w to undertake the programme. This is an important question that not only tests y motivation but also your knowledge of nursing/midwifery and what it entails. You will need to convince the reader that you have some understanding of nursing/midwifery and what nurses/midwives do. Your answer is important and may form a part of the discussion when you are interviewed.

Ethnic origin monitoring forms

Along with the application form you will receive a form that asks questions about your ethnic origin. This is an important form and should be completed and returned with the application form. The United Kingdom is a multicultural society and as a large organization any university or employer has a duty to see that it is attracting a range of students from different ethnic backgrounds. The information contained in this form is confidential and will help the university to discover the facts and publish statistics about the ethnic mix of students applying and taking up places on their programmes. From this information the university can see if it is attracting a range of candidates for its programmes. If the university is not attracting people from a range of ethnic backgrounds or from a specific ethnic group that live locally then the information will help when considering how to attract groups that are under-represented. A university will want to discover why people from a particular ethnic group are not accessing its programmes and then put in measures to improve access.

Health questionnaire

A short health questionnaire is usually also included (however, this may not be sent to candidates until they are offered a place on the programme) with the application form. You will also have a separate envelope in which to return the health questionnaire. The information you provide here is confidential to the occupational health department, therefore you will need to seal the envelope and return it with your application and ethnic monitoring form. Your health questionnaire will then be forwarded by the university admissions office to its occupational health department.

Please be honest about any medical and physical conditions that you may have. Medical conditions and physical disabilities are not necessarily a reason for not accepting a candidate on to a programme, nor are they necessarily a bar to becoming a nurse or midwife. It is important to realize that the occupational health department assesses your health status independently of the academic assessment to determine your suitability as a nursing/midwifery student.

References

The Nursing and Midwifery Council (NMC) requires your university to ensure that applican to nursing and midwifery education are of good health and good character. In orc to demonstrate your good character, and that you have a good employment and/ educational history, you will be asked to provide at least two appropriate referees. Y will need to consider carefully who is best placed to give you such references. It is go practice for you to approach people that you intend to use as a referee beforehand a ascertain their willingness to respond to such requests in a timely manner. It is important be aware that universities place great importance on such references and that your en on to programmes may be delayed if the references are unsatisfactory or are not availab during the application process. It would be a good idea to check with your referees th they have responded to the university's reference request.

Criminal records checks

The Criminal Records Bureau (CRB) is responsible for checking police records and, occasion, information held by the Department of Health (DoH) and the Department Education and Skills (DfES). While there are two CRB checks available (Standard a Enhanced), owing to the privileged nature of healthcare work, and, in particular, workin with vulnerable adults and children, your university is required to obtain an 'Enhanc Disclosure'. Furthermore, as nursing and midwifery is exempted under the Rehabilitati of Offenders Act (ROA) (1974), you are required to disclose all previous convictions a cautions, including those which are 'spent'. However, a criminal conviction or caution not necessarily a bar to undertaking nursing or midwifery education as this can depel on, among other things, the nature of the offence, how long ago it occurred, and wheth or not there have been further offences.

The Enhanced Disclosure is the highest level of background check that can be curren undertaken. It is very important to be honest throughout this process and provide f information when it is needed – failure to do so means jeopardizing your place on tl programme and, indeed, subsequent career. A copy of the Enhanced Disclosure form w be sent to you as well as the university.

Evidence of literacy and numeracy

The NMC requires universities to ensure that all applicants to nursing and midwife programmes have sufficient literacy and numeracy skills to meet both the academic al clinical requirements of the programme. This may mean that you are required to provide evidence of your competency in literacy or numeracy at the point of application or later, at an interview day, where you may be required to sit relevant tests.

At some universities, overseas applicants (i.e. outside of Europe) for nursing and midwifery education may be required to demonstrate their proficiency in English language (listening, reading, writing and speaking) under the International English Language Testing System (IELTS). There is no requirement for European Union (EU) nationals to demonstrate their English language competency in order to register as a Nurse or Midwife. From 1 February 2007, applicants would need to obtain an overall score of at least 7.0. There are many test centres throughout the country (and internationally), and I would advise visiting the IELTS website (www.ielts.org) for further information about the process and how to apply for an IELTS test. Further information on English language proficiency relating to nursing and midwifery can be found at: www.nmc-uk.org/aFrameDisplay.aspx?DocumentID=1843

Accreditation of Prior (Experiential) Learning (AP(E)L)

It may be possible to undertake a shortened nursing programme and here you will need to provide evidence of prior relevant learning (such as qualifications from previous academic courses) or from prior experiential learning (experience resulting from study in a field of health or social care which has been accredited by an approved educational institution). The maximum credit that you could achieve would be one-third of the length of the programme, and you will need to complete a minimum of two years (or 3066 hours). All credit must be supported by authenticated and verified evidence, and mapped against the standards of proficiency of the nursing programme you are applying to (NMC 2004a). If you are awarded such credit, you will be able to join a programme that has already started at a suitable point. This is known as 'advanced standing'. In Midwifery, you can apply for advanced standing *only* if you already have a previous registration in Adult Nursing (Level 1) (NMC 2004b).

This is how it works: collecting academic credits is like putting money into a savings account. You might be saving for a holiday or to buy a car, or you might not be sure what you are going to spend the accumulated money on yet. As with a savings account, you can transfer the credits from one course or university to another. For instance, credits

you gain from studying for a certificate could later count towards a first degree. Differe
universities have different systems to count credits for certificates, diplomas and degre
so you will need to check at the one you are applying to.

If you wish your previous learning to be taken into consideration, you should discuss t
with admission/recruitment staff at the university to which you are applying.

Interview Offer

When you receive a letter offering you an interview, some universities may provide a 't
off' slip for you to complete and return stating whether you will be attending for intervie
If they do not then it is polite to write a short letter or send an email confirming that you
be attending. If you have changed your mind or accepted an offer from another univers
then do write and thank them for the offer of an interview but say that you will not now
attending. You do not have to give a reason but it is helpful to know that you have take
place elsewhere or that since applying you have simply changed your mind.

Having successfully completed the application process and written to accept the offer
an interview you are now in a position to prepare for the interview which will be discuss
in Chapter 6.

Tips

- Consider carefully your choice of programme, the financial implications of study and
  possible impact on your family life before making an application
- Do some homework and find the university that is right for you
- Complete all documentation legibly and honestly
- Consider carefully who is best placed to give you references and approach the
  beforehand
- Consider the possibility of accreditation of prior (experiential) learning (AP(E)L).

Useful Websites

The Website www.nhscareers.nhs.uk/nhs-knowledge_base/data225.ht
provides detailed information regarding NHS bursaries and further information ab

allowances for, for example, dependants, single parents and disabled students. Another useful website is www.nhsgrantsunit.co.uk which has a lot of general information if you are investigating the financial implications of undertaking a nursing or midwifery programme.

References and Further Reading

NMC (2004a) *Standards of Proficiency for Pre-Registration Nursing Education.* London, NMC. Available at: www.nmc-uk.org/aFrameDisplay.aspx?DocumentID=328

NMC (2004b) *Standards of Proficiency for Pre-Registration Midwifery Education.* London, NMC. Available at: www.nmc-uk.org/aFrameDisplay.aspx?DocumentID=171

Chapter 5

The Student with a Disability, Chronic Health or Learning Needs

by Pauline McInnes and Stella Tarantino

In this chapter you will learn:

- **What is a disability?**
- **Why are you and your disability important?**
- **What will student life be like?**
- **What are my rights and responsibilities as a disabled nursing student?**
- **What support can I get before and during my programme?**
- **Who should I tell about my disability?**
- **Tips for success and further reading available.**

Introduction – What is a Disability?

But I am not disabled; surely this chapter isn't for me!

Many people still think of people who are blind, deaf or in a wheelchair when th think about disability, but it's so much wider than that. The Disability Discrimination (DDA) defines disability as 'a physical or mental impairment, which has a substantial a long-term adverse effect on a person's ability to carry out normal day-to-day activit (DDA 1995). Therefore, to be covered by the legislation you should have an impairm that will last for 12 months or more and has a significant impact in your daily life.

Here are some common disabilities among nursing students:

• Specific learning difficulties (Dyslexia or Dyspraxia)
• Asthma
• Epilepsy
• Diabetes
• Mental health difficulties (anxiety, depression, eating disorders)
• Stammer
• Heart condition
• HIV/AIDS
• Sickle cell anaemia
• Visual impairment
• Hearing impairment
• Arthritis
• Cerebral palsy.

This isn't an exhaustive list, but it does give an indication of the varied nature of disabi If you have or know someone who has one of the above impairments or health conditi you really should read this chapter as it might contain some information that is helpfu you or someone you know.

So you have a disability, got the right qualifications, so far so good! What has y educational experience been like up to now – challenge and struggle free? We doubt i you have got as far as thinking about higher education, you must have some stamina a confidence in dealing with 'the system' – possibly some negative experiences or sim just working harder than others to get what you want. It probably wasn't easy. But this ultimately be a valuable asset to you in your healthcare career as the challenges that y may have faced give you an important insight into the needs of others. There are many more challenges that await you in learning to care for other people as well as rewards.

However, a healthcare career could be flexible, fit in with family life, give you great satisfaction to feel you are making a difference and many chances to progress with earnings to match and a passport to success in more ways than one. So, a disability need not be a barrier to a successful and rewarding career. Indeed, one of the recent chief nurses for England tells us that her dyslexia was no barrier to her getting the top job in nursing (Mullally 2005).

Why are You and Your Disability Important?

Why do we want you? You probably know already, you are pretty clued up about living with a disability or health condition and could be a role model for those with less confidence than yourself. You could help to prove that just because you have a disability it doesn't mean that you cannot do the job. You might be a part of a bigger movement to challenge discrimination.

What Will Student Life be Like?

Remember, you won't be alone if you do have a disability. There will be lots of other students (and lecturers!) on your programme with disabilities too. By far the most common one that nursing students have is dyslexia, but it's not the only one. You might want to think about setting up an informal support group for students in your year group so that you can support each other, or find out if one exists to share ideas and problem solve together. You won't always be able to tell which of your colleagues has a disability, so you might want to put up a notice, or send an e-mail to everyone in your year group to find out.

A group like this might help if you find student life a little chaotic, with pressure to join in the socializing, lots of new work, stresses of assignments, no reminders to eat, relax or take medication, and a different level of independence perhaps without usual support from family or partners. By the way, independence doesn't always mean coping with everything on your own! There are lots of reasons why you might suffer minor illness or stress, mixing with new people, starting in your caring role, and probably having to work part time as well. You might have to notice your own changing signs or symptoms, as a new group of

friends/colleagues will not be able to help you pick up the signs and offer you the supp
you may have received from those who have known you for some time. Also, a change
routines might mean that your usual healthy routines might be difficult to maintain.

It is well worth finding out if a nursing or midwifery programme would suit you. Rememb
it is practice focused, and half of your time will be in a clinical setting, where you w
be developing a new range of complex physical and psychological practice skills. T
following list sets out some essentials, and enables a university or yourself to see wheth
it is realistic to think about applying. Best to think ahead and don't set yourself up to fai

What Support Can I Get Before and Durin My Education?

Applicants to nursing or midwifery programmes need to:

- See clearly/communicate clearly, with a reasonable degree of confidence in commu
  cation and interactions
- Have a reasonable degree of manual dexterity/physical ability/strength/stamina
- Have a reasonable degree of accuracy and fluency in written work and numeracy
- If, with reasonable adjustments, you can achieve the above the university should ma
  sure that you can access the same opportunities for learning as those without disabiliti

As a disabled nursing student, there is a much support that you will be able to acce
The first thing to do is start looking at the universities that offer the programme you wa
to study. All universities in the United Kingdom will have someone or a team of peop
who are responsible for providing support to disabled students. Once you have decide
it would be a good idea to get in touch with the Disability Service to find out what sort
support they can provide you with. Many offer prospective students a meeting before
during the application process and this may give you a chance to:

- Meet the people who are going to be supporting you
- Look at the services the university can offer you
- Meet the staff in the library
- Find out if the student accommodation is suitable for you
- Find out if the campus is accessible to you.

Any such meeting will not form part of the selection process. They may also have som
useful booklets so you won't have to try and remember everything.

Finding the Disability Team can sometimes be a challenge as the service may not be well or clearly signposted! If the service is not obvious, the best way to find them is to through the main university's switchboard or search via the university website. The occupational health department or recruitment department at your university may also be able to help with your queries.

The support that you will be entitled to will depend on how your disability affects you, the nature of your programme and, to some extent, the policies and procedures of your university. You may choose to start off with a high level of support and reduce it as you gain confidence, or you may want to try and have as little as possible. Once you are aware of what you are entitled to, it is up to you how you use it. For example, should you have a physical, mental or learning disability, you may need help or adjustments to help support your learning in the university, the skills laboratory or the clinical area. Say you have a hearing impairment, you may need a note taker in class, an amplified stethoscope and/or permission to undertake night duties on a ward where the lights are always on so that you can see to lip-read.

Below are examples of the support that a Disability Service may provide for you:

- Assistance to apply for the Disabled Students Allowance (DSA) and other sources of funding
- Diagnosis of 'Specific Learning Difficulties'
- Organization of alternative examination arrangements
- Liaison with staff members on your programme and throughout the university about your needs
- Setting up non-medical helper support (note takers, dyslexia tuition)
- Provision of loan equipment.

What If I've Never Been Diagnosed as Dyslexic?

There are many students who come to university who do not realize that they have a Specific Learning Difficulty. If you think that you might be one of them after you have enrolled, you should see your Disability Service which will be able to help you to obtain an assessment from an educational psychologist. There could also be funding to pay for these assessments.

Do I Have to Pay for the Support I Need?

Most disabled students who are studying towards a diploma or a degree in nursing entitled to the DSA. For nursing and midwifery students, this allowance is administe through the National Health Service, Student Grants Unit (NHS SGU). If you are a second student (i.e. the NHS trust that you are working for is still employing you while y complete your programme), then you should apply for your DSA through your Lo Education Authority (LEA). It is the DSA that will fund the support you need.

When do I Apply for My Disabled Student Allowance (DSA)?

You should apply for your DSA at the same time that you apply for your bursary and your student loan. If you have already started your programme, you can still apply fo DSA at any time. However, it can take up to four months to receive it, so the earlier y apply the better. You may only get limited support from your university without it.

How do I apply?

To apply for the DSA you need to complete an application form, which can be obtair from the NHS SGU or your LEA. Your university's Disability Service may also hold cop of these forms. Once you have done this, you will need to send it, along with medi evidence of your disability, to the NHS SGU or LEA. Once processed, you will be advisec go and have a Needs Assessment at a recognized Access Centre. It is this assessment t determines what support you will get through the DSA.

What sort of support can I get?

The DSA is not paid to you as a grant and nor is it means tested. Instead, it is an allowar that can be used to purchase the support that you require on your programme as a res of your disability. There are four sections of the DSA.

1. The non-medical helpers' allowance – this pays for human support that you need a result of your disability. For example, note takers, interpreters or study skills tuitio you have a Specific Learning Difficulty.
2. The specialist equipment allowance – this pays for any computer software, hardware specialist furniture or equipment that you need because of your disability. For examp computers, digital recorders, adapted blood pressure readers.

3. The general allowance – this can be used to top up the other two allowances if you run out of money. It may also be used to pay for an Internet connection, extra books or photocopying charges.
4. The travel allowance – this is for students who need to rely on taxi transport because they are unable to drive or to use public transport for all or some of the time.

Once your Needs Assessment has been done, the NHS SGU will write to you to tell you how you should go about organizing your support. The DSA process can seem a very long and daunting one, so it is a good idea to keep in touch with your Disability Service during this time. They will also help you to put the support you receive in place. After this if something is not working for you, then you should go back to them for help or at any time if you feel you are not being treated appropriately, either in university or on your clinical placement.

Support from Student Services/Health Services

For all students, a student services department is a really helpful service to you and can assist with all sorts of advice from money matters to accommodation, from university life to directing you to useful people. Most universities will also have a health centre which will tell you what sort of service they provide, from help in obtaining a GP, stress avoidance or healthy eating sessions, to telling you how to get counselling or survive on a budget.

What are my Rights and Responsibilities as a Disabled Nursing/Midwifery Student

The DDA (1995) ensures that people with disabilities can be protected and have rights under the law which includes when you are a student in further and higher education.

How does the DDA help me?

Under the DDA, universities are required to:

1. Ensure that they do not treat students less favourably, for a reason related to their disability
2. Make reasonable adjustments for students (DDA, 1995).

The legislation relates to all areas of academic study including work placements. The support that you receive through your university, such as alternative examination arrangements and receiving handouts in advance of the class, are all examples of reasonable adjustments, but there are many more. Reasonable adjustments can be made to the environme the way teaching is carried out, policies and written information. The Disability Rig Commission has a lot more information about the DDA and how it affects disabled peo (www.drc.org.uk).

While you are on placement, Part II of the DDA that covers employment also prote you. Therefore, the university and placement provider have a joint responsibility to ens that your needs are met on placement. Some examples of reasonable adjustments placements might include: having a colleague check your spelling, taking regular bre to drink, eat or take medication if necessary, and negotiating attendance. We know t students have been helped to negotiate placement learning after periods when th condition became unstable or if their condition had caused them extra stress, for examp a student with sickle cell anaemia was helped through a stressful period and able reschedule the clinical assessments due.

What if I Think I'm Being Treated Unfairly

If, at any time, you think that you are being treated unfairly because of your disabi or that staff are not making reasonable adjustments for you, you should approach Disability Service of your university. It may just be a matter of one of the Disability Serv staff talking to your personal tutor or programme leader, or being there with you wl you talk to them.

If you feel that neither you nor the Disability Service has been able to resolve the issue th each university will have a complaints procedure that you can go through. Alternativ you can contact the Disability Rights Commission which will be able to advise you ab taking a formal case of discrimination against your university.

Who Should I Tell About My Disability?

It is difficult not to be nervous about saying you have different needs. You may feel t this would lead to misunderstandings or discrimination or you may feel it is unnecess to tell people about your disability because your condition is well controlled. It is up you whom you wish to know about your disability. At university telling people about y disability is known as 'disclosure'. Whom you tell and when you tell them are decisions t only you can make. You can tell one person and ask them to keep it entirely confiden or you can nominate the people you want to know about your disability. You may want people to know what your disability is and what adjustments you are going to need or you may prefer to keep your disability between you, the Occupational Health Adviser and the University Disability Service and just tell other people about your needs.

The benefit of telling people is that they will be able to focus help for you. For example, you may be allowed extra time for your assignments, or your placement mentor may give you extra support in writing up your clinical notes. Universities are expected to make 'anticipatory' reasonable adjustments, for example, providing handouts to all disabled students before the lecture commences. You may need more support than anticipatory adjustments can offer. Finding out how much support your programme tutors offer to all students may help you to decide if you need to disclose to get extra support.

Unfortunately, there are still university staff, medical professionals and indeed patients who will think that, because you are disabled, you should not be on their programme or clinical area. You will need to be prepared to meet people with these attitudes and have some strategies for how you might deal with them and your feelings regarding this.

All learning is about using feedback and sometimes you will hear people say things you don't want to hear. If this happens, the best way to deal with it is to find a way to strengthen your coping methods. If people see that you are motivated and wanting to learn and achieve, you will be assured of a more positive reaction. Being deflated or angry at every negative event or statement will make you defensive and create barriers, and this may be very tiring for you. Think positive and life might begin to become more positive. Celebrate something every day, and don't get frustrated when people don't deliver! Stay calm, be persistent if you really need something or someone to help, and aim for the shortest, easiest route to your destination. Allow the occasional compromise; there doesn't always need to be winners and losers. Challenges can be seen as learning opportunities for all involved. All students can feel excluded or up against the system at some time during their journey, it won't just be you.

Disclosing at Application for Your Nursing/Midwifery Programme

Most application forms for nursing/midwifery programmes will ask if you have a disability. Many universities will also ask this on their enrolment forms. However, universities differ in what they do with this information and who gets to see it. Some will contact you as a result

of a declaration but others may not. So, if you want to be sure that people know ab
your needs, then it might be a good idea to get in touch with the university yourself.

Fitness to Practise

As part of the application process all students must make a declaration that they are
'good health'. This means that you need to be able to practise safely and effectively a
this is not merely about having good health (Skill 2005). Being of 'good health' basic
means that you are capable of meeting the demands of the job without causing harm
yourself or your patients. The Nursing and Midwifery Council (NMC) states that 'Signific
health impairments or disabilities do not, of themselves, preclude people from pract
(Skill 2005).

All students applying to do a nursing/midwifery programme will have to go through Fitn
to Practise assessment. This is done through the university's health department wh
needs to make sure you are fit to join the programme, that you and your patients/clie
are protected and to be sure that you can physically and mentally cope with the demar
of the programme (with reasonable adjustments). This department can also monitor y
progress and be a support throughout the programme if this is appropriate. Often
assessment is just a questionnaire that you need to complete about your health. You
be contacted if there is a concern about anything in this. They may just want to talk to y
about the support that you need, or ask for medical documents or a medical examinati
They might ask you to demonstrate your ability to do certain tasks to assess your capabi
in a clinical placement. If you are concerned about this part of the application, then y
should talk to the university Disability Service or a programme tutor. But remember, it i
your best interests to co-operate with this process.

Disclosing on Placements

Just because you have disclosed a disability to the university does not mean that the s
on your clinical placements will necessarily know about your needs. You may feel that y
don't need any support or that you don't want your clinical colleagues to know about y
disability. However, if you are likely to need extra support, then it might be a good i
to disclose, perhaps just to your ward/unit manager each time you go on placement
you may want to ask for a pre-placement planning meeting. This is where you can m
with someone from your placement and university staff (possibly your link tutor an

member of the Disability Service) to discuss what needs you will have and what reasonable adjustments you might need.

An important focus in clinical placements is being able to apply your academic learning to practice. You will regularly have to adjust to going to different areas about every three months and possibly encounter different challenges each time. The good thing is that you will have mentors in clinical practice out there to help you, but they need to know how they can support your individual needs so you will probably have to remind them of your needs. Make yourself heard, don't worry about asking for help, your mentors are there to do this. It is sometimes useful to be prepared and tell people where they can learn more about your condition. NHS Direct is always a good bet, and there are lots of helpful websites, such as the British Dyslexia Association.

Your Clinical Placement

While on your clinical placement, there may be stresses that you were not prepared for. For example, you will often be undertaking early mornings, late evenings and, sometimes, night shifts. You might also be caring for people who have a similar condition to yourself which may worry or concern you at first. The stresses associated with clinical responsibilities may cause unexpected relapses in your condition. Make sure you seek help if your condition worsens and talk to someone about your concerns.

The health service is a large organization and you will have to fit in somehow. People don't always appear helpful because they are not thinking of just you, especially if they are busy looking after many students or patients/clients. You don't have to be someone you're not but to some extent you have to be prepared to adapt to becoming part of a bigger team, using your strengths, valuing others' strengths and learning from each other.

It is advisable that you tell your clinical mentor about your disability. If, for example, you have epilepsy and occasional night seizures, they might need to know what difficulties you have at night and what might happen if your body clock goes out of 'sync'. If you have dyslexia you may have to think of ways people can check your work as clinical records need to be accurate. If you have Type 1 diabetes, shift patterns might interfere with your normal dietary routine. For example, we know of a situation where a student with diabetes was asked to take a patient to theatre just as she was going for her break. The student was not confident enough to say that she had to have the break otherwise she might

feel ill. Unfortunately she collapsed in the theatre, potentially putting herself and othe
danger.

One of the things that you do not need to disclose to anyone else apart from
occupational health department is your HIV or hepatitis status, as this can be managec
you and Occupational Health taking into full account actual and potential risks. Howe
the University Disability Team may still be able to support you. However, please be aw
that you will not be able to become a midwife if you are HIV positive owing to the na
of the skills involved in delivering babies.

Tips

- Find out about (and contact) the University's Disability Team before applying
- Use University Disability services
- Register with a GP locally
- Take up all the immunizations offered
- Identify a support person from academic or clinical staff
- Share stresses, plan ahead and pace yourself
- Tell room-mates and colleagues contact numbers should you become ill or can't cor
- Aim to keep up healthy lifestyle patterns, balance study, work and play
- It is always your right not to disclose your disability or condition but weigh up the p
  and cons first
- Find out if there is a student support network or others with similar needs. If not, cc
  you start something?

References, Further Reading and Useful Publications

Department for Education and Skills (2006/7) Bridging the Gap: a guide to the Disab
    Students' Allowances (DSAs). In *Higher Education Guide for 2005/06*. London, DfES. (
    guide is produced every year.)
Disability Discrimination Act (1995) Part 4: *Code of Practice for Providers of Post 16 Educa
    and Related Services. 2001*. London, Disability Rights Commission.
Mullally S. (2005) Reflections. *Nursing Standard*, 20(6), 38.
National Bureau for Students with Disabilities (Skill) (2005) *Into Nursing and Midwi*
    Bedford, Newnorth Print Ltd. Available at: www.skill.org.uk/index.asp

Royal College of Nursing (2002) (amended 2006) *Helping Students Get the Best from Their Practice Placements. A Royal College of Nursing Toolkit.* London, RCN.

Royal College of Nursing (2005) *Guidance for Mentors of Student Nurses and Midwives.* London, RCN.

Useful Websites

www.hull.ac.uk/pedds

www.rcn.org.uk/publications for these two publications

Royal College of Nursing website student section: www.rcn.org.uk/students

Skill – National Bureau for Students with Disabilities www.skill.org.uk

Student Finance Direct http://www.direct.gov.uk/StudentFinance

The Disability Rights Commission: www.drc.gov.uk

Chapter 6

The Interview

by David Stroud and Eddie Meyler

This chapter considers:

- **What to do:**
  - **Before the interview**
  - **During the interview**
  - **After the interview**
- **What not to do during the interview**
- **The different type of interview formats you might experience**
- **Typical questions that are asked at interview.**

The interview is the outcome of your decision to embark on a career in nursing or midwif
As the first rung on the ladder leading to registration as a nurse or midwife, the appro
you take to the interviews requires tactical planning if you are to secure a place at
university of your choice.

Preparing for the Interview

An offer to attend for an interview will follow a successful application to your cho
university (or universities), and you will now need to consider how you might best prep

Travel

Try to avoid disasters! Check the venue and how to get there. Plan to arrive early, not
on time, so as to compose yourself before facing the interview panel. Allow time for
unforeseen – such as traffic delays or getting lost. Decide how you will travel to the ver
remembering that most universities have restricted parking. Check the interview locat
carefully as many universities have a number of buildings or campus sites. Besides giv
a bad impression, arriving late can increase your anxiety and prevent you doing your b
If practicable, do a test run of the journey before the interview day.

Personal presentation

What to wear? You do not need a designer suit, but be clean and smart, and dress
way that boosts your confidence. Although there is a move towards informality wit
universities, casual clothes can be perceived negatively by the interview panel.

Checking

Before leaving home, double check that you have everything you have been asked to bri
such as birth certificate, passport, educational qualifications and completed occupatic
health forms if not already sent. Also take a photocopy of your application form
references, as the panel will ask questions related to them. Organize these docume
meticulously, so that you can produce them with ease. Fumbling through a mass of pap
for a particular document is likely to unnerve you, besides giving the impression that
are generally disorganized.

Coping with anxiety

Being interviewed makes everyone but the most accomplished performer nervous. There is a reason for that: it primes you to perform at your best! However, too much anxiety can affect your thinking and behaviour, ruining your performance. There are simple relaxation techniques that can help you. One of the most effective is diaphragmatic breathing. You will need to learn and practise this before the interview. It involves breathing deeply, using your diaphragm (that dome shaped muscle separating your chest cavity from your abdomen) rather than just the muscles of your chest. This naturally leads to deeper, slower breathing that causes you to feel calm and facilitates good speaking. Do it while waiting to be called in, and also during the interview.

Visualization can be very effective in calming your nerves, and there are many books and tapes that show you how to do this. For instance, you can visualize yourself being confident in the interview. Some interviewees imagine a beautiful beach, replete with palm trees, behind the interview panel. Realistic role playing of the interview beforehand, with a sympathetic friend or partner, can also do a lot to steady your nerves and help you to adopt a more positive frame of mind.

Interview Formats

Find out as much as you can about what is expected of you at the interview. The panel will often consist of two to three interviewers, ideally a mix of academics and clinicians. While the academics' focus will be on assessing your ability to complete the programme, the clinician is concerned with your potential ability to be an asset to the nursing or midwifery professions.

In addition to an individual interview, some universities might also require you to be interviewed as part of a group. This often involves a discussion about a topical issue of the day – often health care related. A group discussion can be nerve racking, making you feel like a goldfish in a bowl! So why do they put you through it? Well, it's because there is a need to assess your ability to work as part of a team. You may be given a topic to discuss or a problem to solve. It's important that you contribute without dominating and that you show respect for others. Try not to ramble on, recognize your limitations and make sure what you say is relevant and coherent.

You may be offered a tour of the university on the interview day. Don't forget that thi part of the interview and your reactions and interest may be noticed. Ask any questic that occur to you, for instance, about availability of computers or library opening hours

There might also be a written test, for instance, to assess your literacy or numeracy is common for people to be much better at some basic skills than others. If you ha identified that you need to improve in some area, you can obtain Key Skills books from ye local bookshops. While literacy tests can involve assessing your ability to write coherer in English, numeracy tests are likely to involve your ability to work with numbers. Y may be set a task (or tasks) which might be required to be undertaken under examinat conditions. It might be that you are asked to complete basic calculations and to proble solve with numbers. You might also be asked to complete a written essay on a hea related theme. Increasingly these tests are used to inform a decision about your suitabi to start the programme. If it is felt that you do not have sufficient skills in literacy numeracy to join the programme, it is expected that you will be offered feedback a advice as to how you may improve upon this before applying again.

Engaging with the Interview Panel

An interview is a purposeful conversation, so smile and try to gain rapport with interviewers. Good interviewers will be trying to do the same with you, so you should half-way there. What the interviewers are trying to do is predict the future (i.e. whethe not you are going to be a motivated student and stay for the duration of the programm and they try to do this without prejudice or bias.

Sometimes, panel members might be as nervous as you, and they will certainly warm you if your communication skills help them to feel more at ease! Remember to use gc communication skills, both verbal and non-verbal. Non-verbal skills include maintain an open posture, being relaxed, looking interested, making appropriate eye contact i having an expressive voice. Verbal skills involve answering questions succinctly with digressing, using appropriate language and asking for questions to be repeated or clarif if not understood. The best advice is to be open and honest in the answers that you gi

Things Not to do in an Interview

Here are some things you should not do in an interview (and believe us these h happened!). We would advise that you do not:

- bring your shopping or your children with you (this is not as uncommon as you would imagine!);
- tell the panel that you're in a hurry and will need to leave by at a certain time;
- ask if you can smoke;
- drink alcohol before the interview to calm your nerves;
- attend the interview when you're tired after working night duty;
- turn up late;
- wear a hat or a baseball cap;
- eat or drink, unless refreshments are provided;
- chew gum;
- leave your mobile phone switched on;
- answer your mobile if you have left it on and it rings (switch it off quickly and apologize);
- tell jokes;
- complain about current or previous employers, teachers or past failures;
- be sarcastic;
- pretend to be what you are not;
- try to peek at any notes the interviewers might be making;
- persuade the panel to offer you a place.

In interviewing, as in so many interpersonal situations, it is useful to remember 'primacy' and 'latency' effects. Put simply, what the interviewers may remember most when making their decision is their first and last impression of you.

Possible Questions

The types of questions you might be asked fall into three main categories: closed, open and hypothetical. Closed questions require brief, sometimes monosyllabic answers. Open questions invite longer, more elaborate answers. Hypothetical questions are meant to test how you would react in certain problematic situations. Always aim at being concise, but thorough, in your answers. For the sake of fairness, interviewers try to ask all candidates the same general questions, while remaining flexible enough to probe areas specific to you.

Although interviewers try to refrain from asking inappropriate questions, it is possible that they may do so innocently. The question could be to do with issues such as marriage, childcare arrangements, sexuality, race, gender, or political or religious beliefs. These questions should not be the concern of the interview panel as this may compromise equal

opportunities. It will be to your credit if you handle the question tactfully and with[ ]
getting angry. You might like to calmly say something like 'I'm not sure how I fee[ ]
answering that question'. This would give the interviewer the opportunity to reconsi[ ]
their question, perhaps rewording it or dropping it altogether.

Some of the questions frequently asked are:

Why have you chosen to apply for the programme?

Here, your answer should be an honest appreciation of the issues that have inspi[ ]
you to enter nursing or midwifery. Try to say something about you as a person t[ ]
also reflects your understanding of nursing or midwifery. You should also be clear ab[ ]
the reason for choosing either midwifery or a particular branch of nursing (adult, ch[ ]
learning disabilities and mental health). However, it is not always clear to the interv[ ]
panel why a prospective student has chosen a particular programme. Sometimes i[ ]
evident that the student has not thought through their decision in respect of their fut[ ]
career. This will not help you to secure a place on the programme! So you should read[ ]
the literature that is sent to you and also get as much information as you can from ot[ ]
sources.

If your intended career move is from a desk job to nursing or midwifery, try to sh[ ]
how your previous skills and knowledge are transferable. Most jobs require the skill[ ]
communication, problem solving and personal management. Emphasize how your val[ ]
are manifested in such behaviours as team working, good timekeeping and attention[ ]
detail.

Tell us a little about yourself

This is an invitation for you to sell yourself. Tell the panel about being a school prefect, ab[ ]
winning a prize, about captaining a sports team, about any extra-curricular activity. T[ ]
about any voluntary or community work you've been involved in. This is an opportun[ ]
to demonstrate that you have desirable qualities such as leadership, determination a[ ]
altruism.

The panel will already have an impression of you from your application form and y[ ]
presentation, so don't describe yourself as a totally different person. Describe yoursel[ ]
you are, not as you would like to be!

Tell me about your hobbies or interests

This question is a potential minefield. There is a temptation to give an answer that you believe will impress the panel, such as 'reading'. They will then ask what you read, and you'll reply, 'Nursing books and articles'. Now you are bound to be asked what book you are reading currently and what interesting article you have read recently. So be prepared to give precise answers about your reading. If you read fiction for relaxation, fine, just say so. Some candidates mention that they do voluntary work associated with their spiritual beliefs or for particular charities – do mention this as it demonstrates a commitment to, and a concern for the welfare of, others which is an essential feature of any healthcare professional.

How do you promote your own health?

The panel want to know if you have a healthy balance of intellectual and physical activity, and they will be impressed by such a lifestyle. Health promotion is not only about how you look after your body, but also your mind! So, mention anything that helps you to keep fit, but also anything you do to cope with the stress and strains of life – such as gardening. Again, try not to impress the panel by saying that you regularly run marathons when it is clear you don't! Be honest here – don't be afraid to say you watch TV or go to the pub, too!

What are your strengths and weaknesses?

Many candidates find this a difficult question, so it is worth brainstorming a list of these before the interview, or even asking a friend to give you honest feedback. Some strengths might be: caring, works well in a team, reliable. Weaknesses might be more difficult, but remember that the panel is not looking for perfection – they are looking for self-awareness. Some strengths can be disguised as weaknesses, such as: 'Sometimes I work so hard that I don't take time for relaxation', 'I tend to put everyone else's needs before my own' or, 'I find it difficult to say no when people ask me for favours'. Although you should answer these questions honestly, don't wallow in your shortcomings!

What work experience have you had?

Although this will be on your application form, you will be asked to enlarge on it. It is important to emphasize transferable skills and knowledge. If, for example, you are working in a supermarket, talk about your ability to communicate with the public and how you can keep calm in challenging situations. Being a healthcare assistant in a hospital gives you

the opportunity to show you understand the healthcare system in the United Kingdo
If there are gaps in your work record you should be ready to explain this in a posit
way – time off to study, travel or to raise a family.

What academic experience do you have?

Again, this will be on your application form. Even if your highest qualification is
'Access to Nursing' course, be proud of your achievement. Your life experience is jus
valuable; there is no substitute for learning from experience. Be open about any acade
shortcomings. If your science or essay writing is weak, acknowledge it and convince
panel that you are prepared to work hard to improve it. If you were called for intervi
you must have at least met the minimal academic requirements. Rather than a candid
who tries to show that they are perfect, the panel prefers an individual who says, 'I kno
need to improve'. Try to strike a balance between boasting and being over-modest!

If you have a degree or are academically above the entry requirements, do not assume t
your selection is automatic. It is also essential that you demonstrate that you are self-aw
and that you can work as part of a team. It is also helpful to show that you'll be prepa
to share your knowledge and experience with other students.

Would you like to ask us anything?

Take the opportunity to ask any questions you might have, such as those about program
start dates, holiday entitlements, changing branch of nursing during the programm
uniform allowance, availability of accommodation or when you'll know if you've be
successful. Some students might ask the interview panel their opinions about the imp
of the programme on family life. However, although this is an era of equal opportunit
the panel may be concerned if you have not already considered the personal dema
nursing or midwifery education will have on you.

Most application forms ask if you have any special learning needs, such as dysle
(difficulties with recognizing words) or dyscalculia (difficulties with recognizing numbe
You should openly acknowledge any disability because universities have a legal obligat
to provide such students with support and facilities to enable them to succeed (
Chapter 5).

Tips

- Be prepared, be confident and try to do your best
- Check the interview time, date and venue
- Check your documentation prior to setting off for the interview
- Try to relax during the interview
- Answer the interview panel's questions openly and honestly
- List any questions that you would like the panel to answer
- Remind yourself that, just as you would like a place on the programme, the nursing and midwifery professions need good practitioners and the university needs enthusiastic students.

Section 2

Developing Your Academic Skills

Nursing and Midwifery education comprises both theoretical and practical elements. Throughout your education you will be required to demonstrate your skills in both these areas. It is fair to say that the theoretical component of the programme often poses the most challenges for students and this is perfectly understandable for reasons discussed in Section 1.

In this section, we turn our attention to helping you to meet the theoretical requireme of the programme – how to, in other words, develop academic skills. As the authors in section will highlight, these skills are essential not only to help you complete the necess assessments for the programme, but will help you to develop your knowledge base the skills of analysis so essential for practice in complex modern healthcare situations.

Issues that are covered here include helping you to use electronic and library resource develop your knowledge base and understanding of healthcare issues; how to develor analytical approach as a precursor to effectively critiquing the healthcare literature; hov organize, plan and write your assessments in an academic way, including how to refere your work; and how to fully utilize current and previous feedback in order to improve develop your theoretical work.

We would suggest that you read all these chapters together before setting out to comp your academic task.

Chapter 7

Using Information Technology

by Anthony Meyler

In this chapter you will learn about:

- **How to get the best out of technology and ideas about purchasing equipment**
- **How to avoid the common disasters that beset students, such as failing to back up and look after your electronic data**
- **How to save work and protection from viruses and other threats**
- **How to do Internet searches for relevant websites.**

Introduction

This chapter will make the following assumptions:

- You have used a version of Microsoft Windows and Microsoft Office within the last yea
- You have, or will have, Internet access
- You will not be using an Apple Mac computer.

Information Technology (IT) is becoming increasingly important in health care (and inde healthcare education) and it is essential, therefore, that you become familiar with tl basics. IT has impacted industry and the public sector for over a decade and its effect relentless. It is a revolution the likes of which we have never seen before.

Everyone comes to healthcare education with different levels of proficiency, but everyor should aim to become at least competent in using IT during their course. Developing yo competence involves you developing your confidence and the best tactic here is to give a go! You are not going to 'break' the Internet or wipe your computer of all data becau you have pressed the wrong button and always remember in the worst case scenario the is always the 'off' button! You will learn best by trial and error – press a button see what does! And while there are some really excellent courses that you could attend and boo that you could buy, nothing beats learning by interacting directly with your computer ar its software.

This chapter is primarily aimed at those of you who might be daunted by terminology ar the prospect of using IT; after reading it I hope that everyone will feel able to use IT support their studies. That is, I will try to offer you a pathway to becoming competent using your computer so that you will (hopefully) see it as more than a mess of wires ar lights in the corner of your room!

The Health Service of the Future?

Here is a version of the future and I will let you decide if it is plausible or just scien fiction . . .

It starts with an online database called 'Spine' that will contain all patient records fro home addresses to allergies. You can visit your local doctor and receive an online heal examination. It will be possible to talk to a physician around the clock and schedu appointments to fit into your day. Patients would not only receive their National Health Service (NHS) number but also a biometric security pass to access the NHS superhighway information service.

So how will you fit into this bigger picture? It may be that in the not too distant future your role may be not only to offer direct clinical care but also to respond to electronic queries from members of the public or to attend virtual ward rounds or other multiprofessional meetings. The efficiency of future healthcare services will be directly related to the skills and abilities of staff who provide the care, and for that reason becoming skilled in using IT will ensure your future and afford you the necessary skills to move with the times.

How plausible is this? Well these are the Government's stated plans – if you would like to know more, then further information about the 'National Programme for IT in the NHS' (including 'Spine') can be found at: www.connectingforhealth.nhs.uk

The University of the Future?

One of the ways in which you will be prepared for using IT in your clinical practice will be by using online learning resources at your university. This can be in the form of reference materials, quizzes, online chats with other students, or 'virtual' tutorials.

Increasingly, your courses and programmes will involve 'blended learning'. That is, a theme or issue which was discussed in a lecture or tutorials is further developed by reading online materials or undertaking structured activities via an electronic portal, such as 'Blackboard'.

Sometimes, online learning can even replace many of the teaching activities which involve direct contact with tutors (save for tutorials), requiring you to become more self-sufficient and taking control for your own learning. This is most common with 'distance learning' courses or programmes, such as those offered with great success by the Open University.

Jargon Busting

First things first. Let's try to clarify some of the strange terms and abbreviations that you are likely to encounter:

Software – programmes and applications that allow you to do things with your computer, such as word processing and playing games

Software suite – a combination of programmes that allow you to undertake different tas
for example, Microsoft Office, Norton SystemWorks

Hardware – simply put, hardware is anything that can be touched, so this would inclu
the base unit, printers, mouse and so forth

USB – that is, 'Universal Serial Bus'. This is a very common type of connection for swif
and easily connecting a wide variety of hardware to your computer, such as printe
and external storage devices

URL – that is, 'Uniform Resource Locator'. Simply, this is the web address of the site you a
looking for, for example, `www.nmc-uk.org`

Geeky – an adjective describing the tendency to become infatuated with computers.

It's a Set Up!

Buying a computer

Before you buy, decide upon a budget. But consider this: whatever you buy will be o
of date within two years! Therefore by keeping to a mid-range quality machine it will
possible to save some cash and maintain reliability while having enough of the toys (su
as digital cameras, scanners, etc.) that come with your computer to be fashionably 'geek

Getting to know you

Setting up your computer (from the box) is usually the first step in building this importa
relationship. It is vital that you get this first step right, so take your time and read
instructions available before assembling anything! At this point, you will be surrounded
wires, boxes and assorted strange looking things that bear little or no resemblance to t
picture on the box. And unless the people you bought it from are environmentally awa
enough packaging to melt a small glacier. This is normal and if you find yourself enjoyi
all this you, too, are becoming 'geeky'.

On most new computers a colour coded scheme is used to provide even more help wh
putting everything together. A small piece of advice – if you have to force a connector
then this is a bad sign. It means you have either got the wrong connection, have position
it incorrectly, or are colour blind.

Lastly, after you have double checked your connections take a deep breath, press t
power button, and turn it on. It is likely that you will have a few on screen questions wh
the various installed pieces of software start for the first time. I would make a note of yo
responses for future reference in case you have to phone a manufacturer with a query.

Getting connected

The final and most crucial step is to get connected to the Internet (either via a 'dial-up' connection or now more commonly 'broadband'). To gain access to the Internet you will need an Internet Service Provider (or 'ISP'). There are many ISPs, and at the time of writing this I counted at least 12, one of which also provided broadband via a satellite (using microwaves for the technically minded).

Security

Now we have to protect your valuable assets, and this is where virus protection is so important. The most important part of having virus protection is ensuring that it is updated regularly. Sadly, there are many viruses on the Internet (with new ones being developed all the time) that vary in lethality – some can cause grave damage to your computer, some are merely annoying. For example, the virus Blaster caused computers to shut down every few minutes.

At one time, we used to associate viruses with maliciously damaging your computer. Today, we find an increasing number of programs that will 'spy' on you and the personal information on your computer. So, if you are buying an anti-virus product, it will be worth while ensuring that it has the full range of software to protect your personal information.

An important rule of thumb in protecting your computer from viruses and 'spyware' is this: If you do not trust the source of the information then reject it. This applies to messages, files, disks – anything that might come into contact with your precious computer. Furthermore, if you are online *never give out any information about yourself without fully trusting the system or person that has made the request*. If you decide to purchase books online ensure that you only do so from a website that is secure and reputable.

The computer is my friend!

It is important to familiarize yourself with the installed software and all the additional equipment. It is likely that your computer will have a selection of software that can produce letters, spreadsheets, databases, plus other software that will help you with multimedia (audio and visual) and virus protection. You might also have a printer, scanner, DVD/CD-writers, camera, plus USB storage devices. Some of the instruction books that come with this software can be weighty tomes, but do try to read at least the summary to get a broad instructional overview.

You will certainly need a printer as we are still a few years away from completely abandoni
hard copies of files. The printer can be low maintenance (basic output quality and lo
cost, such as an inkjet printer) or high maintenance (expensive to buy and run, and oft
attention seeking but with superb output quality, such as laser printers). An importa
piece of advice when it comes to printers is to make sure your paper is suitable to use
your printer, is new and crisp and never, ever try to rush it! Use a minimum paper weig
of 80 g with your printer – 90 g is even better.

I Got You Back

Backing up, saving and safely storing your work is absolutely vital. There are some extreme
fancy pieces of software that will make sure that you can re-animate your computer af
the most catastrophic disasters. These tend to be more complex and time consumi
but they are worth the effort. I will concentrate on only a couple of basic and foolpro
methods of making sure that your data remain safe and usable.

Storing your work

Try not to rely only on the hard drive of your computer to store your valuable wo
Invest in a DVD recorder – a good quality one is inexpensive today and should include t
necessary software. Do not try to fit this if you are in any doubt as this does require son
technical know-how. In fact, some shops will offer to fit the unit for a small charge. B
some recordable DVDs, watch out for speeds and try and match it to the speed of yo
DVD unit. DVDs should stay at home in a safe place and out of direct sunlight. Try not
use them as a coaster. However, this method is not a 100% safe as errors can occur wh
writing or the disk may contain imperfections.

Buying USB storage

So Plan B, buy a USB storage device as another way of backing up your work! It is possi
to lose either or both your DVD and USB copy so be careful! The USB device is design
to be robust and mobile; it may even join you on a workout at the gym. There are ma
inventive ways to avoid losing your USB device; some include attaching it to the car ke
while some people attach it to the neck lanyard which also holds your photo ID card.

Buying your USB storage device (sometimes known as 'pen drive' or 'flash drive') is I
buying a cup of coffee. You might go to a coffee shop with the intention of buying

straightforward 'Americana' with milk and two sugars but end up with the triple vanilla latte with whipped cream and a flake. Like a cup of coffee, the USB storage device can come in many different shapes, sizes and with different extras. They have officially replaced the floppy disk as a method for transporting data. Unlike the floppy disk, and unlike a cup of coffee for that matter, USB storage devices come in different capacities with fast transfer speeds. It is possible to buy a basic 128 MB USB drive for about £10.00 (which is probably all you need for your course). If money is no object, an 80-GB (80 000-MB!) device will play music, video, and TV programmes, as well as any important files and documents, and will probably cost in excess of £200 (this is your triple vanilla latte!).

Caught in a Net?

In this section, I will take you through some key things to remember when attempting to find that useful piece of information or website on the Internet (Chapter 8 will offer advice on finding academic literature using health-related databases).

How to search on the Internet

Turn the computer on and find the program that browses the Internet. There are a few available but the most common program is Microsoft's 'Internet Explorer'. The layout of these programs is the same, in that commonly used buttons will be large and across the top of the screen on the 'toolbar'. These are your shortcut buttons that give you control when you are searching online.

There are many search engines that you might use to locate useful healthcare information and websites on the Internet. For example, Google (www.google.co.uk) and Yahoo! (www.yahoo.co.uk) are commonly used, reliable Internet search engines. When on the search engine's home page, you will find a box, clearly marked, into which you type key words that you wish to explore. Any useful website addresses (technically their URL) you find should be put into your 'favourites' menu so that you can access them without having to repeat searches unnecessarily.

You might also wish to use specific subject gateways, such as Intute (www.intute.ac.uk/healthandlifesciences/nursing/) to help you locate quality information from the Internet. Intute is an excellent, free online service which provides access to Internet web resources for education and research, which are selected and evaluated for quality by subject specialists. This can be more useful than conducting searches on one of

the general search engines and having to sift through the large number of hits you h
found, which are more helpful to another profession or discipline. You should also get i
the habit of evaluating the quality of what you find from the Internet. Not everything y
find on the Internet is of an academic standard suitable for an assignment!

Getting quality results

Unless you choose your words carefully, you will find that your search engine will give y
more results (often called 'hits') than you can reasonably cope with. So, the first step
obtaining a manageable number of hits is choosing your words wisely. This is the first s
in the process known as 'filtering'.

Choosing your words carefully will save you time by reducing the number of results
hits but will also improve the quality of the information that you will obtain. A go
quality search engine will provide you with advanced search features to strengthen y
searching, such as confining your search to particular languages. This can be found un
the 'advanced search' option.

How to search strongly

A quality search is a 'strong' search. By this, I mean that you obtain a manageable num
of hits and those that are most useful for your purposes, simply by using quote marks a
a minus symbol!

So, let's start with a weak search and build up our strength! If you type

   primary health care

(without the quote marks) into Google, at the time of writing you will obtain 237 000
hits! That is, 237 000 000 pages on websites that contain the words 'primary', 'health' a
'care'.

However, if you typed:

   'primary health care'

(note the quote marks) Google will give you 10 800 000 hits. In search terms the qu
marks mean 'search only this'. However, I'm sure you will agree this is still too m
websites to sift through!

Now, assume you don't want to be sold any products relating to primary health care (and remember the Internet is one big market place!). That is, you will need to take out all websites that are trying to sell you something, or to entice you with special offers, then you could remove references to this. So, if you were to type in:

'primary health care' – special offer

(i.e. if you put a minus sign before the term or phrase you wish to exclude) you will find that your hits have been dramatically reduced (try it and see!).

So now let's try for a very strong search. Try this for yourself and see how these simple techniques can change your life! Assume that you are interested in primary mental health nursing care in the NHS, not in the United States or Europe, and still didn't want to be sold anything. Type in:

'primary health care' 'NHS' 'mental health' 'nursing' – special offer – USA – Europe

How many hits do you have now?

Web Based E-Mail Account – Electronic M@IL

What is a web based e-mail account? It is an e-mail account that you can access from any computer that has an Internet connection. You will usually have to visit the website and sign up to its e-mail services and from that point on whenever you wish to check your e-mail, it is just a matter of visiting that site and logging on with a username and password. Most Internet providers will offer this service plus there are specialist websites that offer only this service, it is generally a 'free' service so choose one with lots of space on offer.

Why do I need a personal web based e-mail account? Well, it will provide you with two essential things: a way of corresponding with others on the Internet and a location on the Internet for storage (it will depend on the size of your mailbox). I am now going to give you a great little tip. Send your work to yourself! Type in your personal e-mail address (say from your university e-mail account) then attach the document, with a subject and message. Now press send and it arrives in your inbox ready for you to action. You now have a number of copies of your valuable work – one on your USB storage device, a DVD back up, a copy at your personal web based e-mail account, and the copy that is on the computer!

Living with a Computer

The future of the computer within the home environment has been changed and redefine by technological advancements in software (programs) and hardware (equipment), an broadband Internet. Instead of simply putting together basic documents and formulatii calculations, the computer can now entertain the kids, make long distance phone cal produce video, and synchronize with PDAs (personal data appliances) and mobile phone

The day-to-day use of your computer will involve very little maintenance, save for regul dusting and the occasional hiccup when you have to change the printer cartridge. Howeve living with a computer can present many problems particularly when you have a partn or a family to share it with. You may well find that you will need to negotiate access the computer, and the amount of time you spend on it. Consider the time of day you ca dedicate to your research and coursework requirements and balance this against everyor else who wants a piece of the computer.

You will also need to take steps in case your work is accidentally deleted or moved k another person who has access to your computer. This also applies if you are working or computer in your university's library or an Internet cafe, and be aware that if your work taken by another, it can be difficult for you to prove your authorship. So, always rememb to log out and adopt wise saving and back-up practices to protect your hard work!

Efficient use of the computer can mean different things but I would like to focus on essa writing and research. I will make one single recommendation and that is to learn to 'touc type'. I know of several software packages available on the Internet and in computer sho| that will teach you how to type. It would be worth while visiting a local college or furth education establishment to investigate a keyboarding course. Whether you choose th software or a dedicated course it will still require some time and commitment and it is skill borne of repetition.

You will need to familiarize yourself with the keyboard layout by conditioning ar instinctively reaching for the correct key and not looking for it. I have mentioned repetitio and I feel it prudent to point out that poor posture and overuse of the keyboard ca severely affect the body, joints and even your vision. It is always wise to have a quic check of current guidelines for use of a computer, however, like most thought intensiv and repetitive activities it is always worth getting regular breaks in, not too regul though!

Tips

- When buying a computer, choose one that is mid-priced and consider after sales support
- Sign yourself up for free electronic e-mail
- Don't be afraid – press buttons and see what happens
- Be careful about taking breaks while using your computer, and gently mobilize your arms and neck to avoid injuries
- Be mindful that you might have to share your computer
- Adopt good practices when it comes to backing up and saving your work
- Learn to touch type!

Chapter 8

Getting the Most From Your Library

by Pam Louison

In this chapter you will learn about:

- **The practicalities of using a library**

- **How to become information literate**

- **How to search for literature using library catalogues and electronic databases**

- **What to do if it all goes wrong.**

Introduction

Using today's libraries means being 'information literate'. This is the ability to obtain a
use the information you need to help you complete your programme of study; to locat
efficiently and effectively; and also being able to evaluate and reference it correctly. T
may seem daunting when you are beginning your programme, but there are techniqu
you can use to help you acquire the skills you need, and always remember that help
available within the library. It is also important to keep in mind that in order to deve
any new skills, you need to practise using them. The more you use those skills for your o
personal development, the more efficient and effective library user you will be.

The majority of libraries contain a mixture of print and electronic sources of informati
so to use the library most productively you will need to have an awareness of how to u
a computer.

Practicalities of Using a Library

There are some practical things that you need to know when using the library. While so
may seem obvious, they are, however, the simple things that always seem to be forgott

Location and layout of your library

Start off by finding out where your library is! Sounds simple, but if you are on a multi-
university that has more than one library, you may find books related to your program
housed on several sites. Also, find out when the library is open – libraries are often op
out of hours (i.e. before 9 a.m. and after 5 p.m.) and sometimes over the weekend.

Familiarize yourself with the layout of the library. Where are the photocopiers? How
they work – by cash or card? Most obvious of all, where do you need to place the origi
on the plate in order to photocopy an item and what copy output can you underta
single sided only, double sided, reduction and enlarging of images or texts on to pape
acetate? If you have to pay for your photocopying, trial and error can be an expensive w
of obtaining a readable copy!

Be aware of how the books and journals are arranged – is everything related to y
subject on one floor or is it spread over several floors? Are there separate collections
the books, journals and government reports? If relevant books are available across

university campus, find out how you request items from other parts of the university campus, and how long it takes. You might also have access to other university libraries and your university may be a member of several co-operative schemes that will enable you to access a wider range of resources, as well as those available where you are studying.

Available services

Next, look at the services available. What is available and how do you access them? Do you need usernames and passwords to access all or some of the services available to you, and if so, how do you go about acquiring them? Do you need to create them yourself or are they created for you? If they are created for you, how do you access them? An important point is this: remember to note down any usernames, passwords and PIN numbers you create (and the applications to which they belong), and keep them safe.

Remote access

You will be expected to use a range of resources to complete your assignments and projects, so find out if the main sources of information are available electronically as well as in printed format within the library, and if you can access them remotely (i.e. from another computer outside of the library). That is, you may not always need to physically visit the library all the time in order to access resources. You may also be able to check out what is available from the library via the Internet. If you are on a distance learning programme, on a clinical placement or on a part-time programme, you will find it useful to know what library services you can access remotely. You may find it useful to draw up a checklist of what's available and how it can be accessed. Bookmark or add websites to your favourites on your own computer so that you can access them easily.

Loans

When you are considering borrowing material, it is important to be aware of, and to distinguish between, the types of books and other literature available within the library. For example, what's available for a long loan, short loan or reference only? There will be markings on the books to enable you to denote the status of items available within the library.

You also need to know how many items you can borrow at any one time and if renewals are allowed on the items you have borrowed. Please remember to look at the date stamp of the items you have borrowed, and if necessary make a note of it to remind you when

they need to be returned or renewed. Aim to use items you have borrowed within the lo
period, just in case they have been reserved and remember that you will still be expect
to return items when you are out on placement.

If you are looking for a particular article from a journal that the university does not sto
then, usually for a small fee, your librarian will be able to order this for you from anotl
library. Likewise, if an essential book is not stocked within your library, your librarian v
be able to request it from another library for you.

Finally, what might happen if everything on your reading list is out on loan? Well, hav
think about what other titles you can look for and seek help from your librarian if you ;
not sure what alternatives there might be for your information need. The librarian can he
you find alternative sources while you wait for the item you require to be returned fro
loan.

Renewals

To avoid hefty penalty fines for not returning the books on time, it is worth wh
familiarising yourself with the methods available for you to renew items. Can you ren
items over the Internet, on the phone in or outside of library hours, or do they have to
renewed in person? Make use of any electronic or telephone renewal system available
items cannot be renewed, or if you cannot return the item to your home site, are you a
to return it to one of the other campus sites, or, if necessary, post it back?

Searching for Information

The process of searching the library catalogue, an electronic database, or a range of ot
information sources, is referred to as 'literature searching'. It is, in fact, a search for
healthcare literature you need to enable you to back up your knowledge and argume
in your academic and practice assessments. To succeed in your studies you will need
get into the habit of undertaking a search whenever you need information.

Using the library catalogue

It is of vital importance that you learn how to use the library catalogue to find healthc
literature. It is less time consuming to master using the catalogue than to wander arou
the library in the hope that you will spot the book you wanted to borrow! Not only will
catalogue let you see what is available, it will let you know what is out on loan, and whe

is due for return. You should also be able to reserve items that are out on loan if you need to read them. You may also be able to access your own borrower record, to check what you have out on loan and renew items.

The catalogue will let you see the full range of learning resources available to you in terms of books, journal titles, CDs or DVDs. Many catalogues also link to the reading lists given to you, so knowing how to use the catalogue should be viewed as a necessity rather than a chore.

As part of your induction and orientation to your library you should receive a demonstration as to how the catalogue works. If you find the task daunting, use the catalogue to carry out one task at a time but use it often so that you can build up your skills. You don't need to master how to use the catalogue in one day, but you should know how it works by the time you move on to the next module in your programme.

To start with, use the reading lists or handouts you receive as part of your programme to search the catalogue using an author and title, author, or keyword (i.e. a topic or subject). Familiarize yourself with the layout of the catalogue screen and see what information you need to type in, and what you need to click on in order to locate the shelf number of the information you are looking for.

Electronic health databases

To find online journal articles, you will need to access an appropriate electronic database. There are many such databases. Some of the more common ones that you may come across are:

- BNI (British Nursing Index)
- CINAHL (Cumulative Index to Nursing and Allied Health Literature)
- Cochrane Library (a huge database which collates reliable evidence on the effects of health care).

Accessing these databases is straightforward, usually via 'resources' such as OVID or EBSCOhost EJS. Using a gateway service, such as 'Athens' (a secure access management for UK Education and Health sectors), means that all your resources can be found quickly and easily. To use Athens you will need a password and a username – usually supplied by your library. Indeed, many universities will set this up for you as part of the enrolment process to your programme.

While this may seem daunting, it is a lot easier to use one of these databases than to
through by hand a number of journals that are found in your library. Equally, if you
looking for something specific, you may find useful information in a journal that is
one that seems relevant to your subject area or speciality. Sure, you may stumble acr
something useful and interesting while hand searching, but it does save time learning h
to use a database efficiently.

Principles of searching

The principles of searching databases include: thinking of keywords and phrases relat
to the subject or topic, having alternative keywords and phrases, being aware of w
sources of information are available for the subject, using 'limiters' (discussed later in
chapter) to obtain a manageable number of items, analysing and evaluating what you f
and writing up what you find.

When searching, remember to note down all the details of the literature you wish to use
you will need to ensure that this is referenced fully and accurately. There's nothing wo
than writing up an assignment, and realizing that you have not recorded the informat
needed to cite details correctly!

Searching electronic databases

Some of the skills you have learnt when accessing information via the library catalo
can equally be applied to finding information on an electronic database. Obtain
information via health databases (such as research articles contained within journal:
other periodicals) is actually quite straightforward and there are a number of way
which you can search a database. The database will ask you to provide details of
words, phrase, subject heading, authors and so forth that are the main focus of your qu
However, if you have a specific article in mind, you can also use the database to search
information by a particular author or article title, and you can target a search at a partic
journal. Databases are also useful if you need to check a reference given to you that r
be inaccurate.

So, to summarize, this is how it works (I am assuming that you will be using the 'Athe
gateway service).

1. The quickest way and most efficient way of using 'Athens' is to go directly to the web
    (www.athens.ac.uk). However, if you are using a computer within the univer

library, you might find a quick link on the 'desktop' to the Athens site. Occasionally, a university might require you to access Athens via its own 'portal'.

2. Click on the 'My Athens' tab. (Sometimes you will need to take a minute or two to locate the buttons you need on web pages.)
3. You will then be directed to the page where you need to 'Log on'. Type into the appropriate sections your username and password.
4. Once you are successfully logged in, you will be directed to the 'MyAthens' homepage. Click the 'Resources' button.
5. You will be directed to the 'List of Resources' page. Click on the resource you wish to use (common resources in health care are OVID Online, EBSCOhost EJS and Ingenta Select).
6. In your resource, select the database(s) that you wish to search (e.g. CINAHL, Cochrane). You will then be directed to the main search page.
7. Search your chosen database(s) for the literature by using keyword phrase, subject heading, authors and so forth.

Improving your searching

One of the common problems when searching databases is the high number of results (or 'hits') that you might obtain. For example, let's assume that you wish to find all literature relating to 'health promotion'. If you are using the CINAHL database, at the time of writing you will find 11 234 research articles and other literature if you use 'health promotion' as your key words. It would take many hours to sift through these results!

Remember the quality of the information you get out of the database is dependent on the information you put in. The database cannot give you the answers on its own so you have to think of the key words and tell it what you are after! Your induction to the library should include an introduction to literature searching, and also how to conduct a search using an appropriate database. In order to carry out an efficient search, you need to be aware of the stages involved. The literature search strategy you devise should be formulated at the very beginning of your search, before you do anything (for further information on developing an analytical approach please see chapter 9; for suggestions on developing a literature searching strategy please see chapter 10; and see chapter 11 for some information on planning your theoretical assessments).

Be sure that you understand what you are looking for. You could go through the whole process of searching only to realize at the end that you were on the wrong track, and should have been looking for something entirely different. Equally, you may have very clear ideas of what information you want to retrieve, only to be frustrated when searching because whatever keyword or phrase you typed in keeps coming up with no results.

Reducing the number of 'hits'

In addition to being specific regarding what information you are wishing to find, databa
can help you to limit the 'hits' by allowing you to confine your search to within cer
parameters. For example, your search can be restricted to a certain year of publication
between two dates; whether or not you want a full text copy of any article; and whet
you want publications in English only.

Some online resources, such as OVID, allow you to search more than one database a
time. The potential problem here is that you might find that each database contains
same articles! If this is the case you can usually delete these duplications which will red
the number of 'hits'.

On your nursing/midwifery programme you should receive instruction on how to acc
information appropriate databases, but if you are in any doubt then do speak to y
librarian. You can also obtain further information about searching healthcare databa
by consulting the relevant 'help' page for your chosen database.

What to do if it All Goes Wrong

Whilst you are expected to acquire the skills for using the library independently, do
forget that you do have access to a librarian and others in the library who are there to h
you. Please don't wait until the morning before your assignment is due to seek help a
assistance! Neither should you be embarrassed to approach your librarian or membe
the library if you have already received information regarding the service you want to u
Using the library and database searching can be difficult to grasp all at once. There is a
to take in. It is unrealistic to assume that you will know everything after receiving a b
induction.

You should have an opportunity to reflect on your knowledge and skills as you progr
throughout your programme. Don't forget the library in this reflection process a
remember that you need to prepare your search before you sit down at the database
even before you use the library. Keep in mind the purpose of why you are looking
information, what information you are trying to find, how you are going to search for
information you need, where you can look for the information you want, and if you
stuck whom you can consult for help.

Tips

- Do speak to your librarian if you need help or advice regarding accessing information
- Master the essential skills required to use the library effectively – it will help you to prepare for lifelong learning and assist in your personal and professional development throughout your career
- Invest some time in learning how to use online databases.

Chapter 9

Becoming Analytical

by Deirdre Kelley-Patterson

This chapter considers:

- **What analytical thinking really means**
- **How you can develop deep approaches to learning and understanding (in the classroom and in the practice environment)**
- **What you do in the face of uncertainty.**

Introduction

When you start your programme you will probably find that you have strayed int[o] rule-bound world with clear statements about what you must and must not do. Such ru[les] are often important to ensure that you, your colleagues, your patients and the public [are] safe. However, sometimes it can be unclear what purpose some rules seem to serve a[nd] sometimes rules develop as a result of custom or habit! The problem with rules is t[hat] they might be adopted and followed without thought – that is, rules might well constr[ain] people's ability to make decisions and to develop new and innovative ways of working[.]

As your course progresses and as you gain experience in a range of practice environme[nts] you will be faced with the need to make decisions and to decide for yourself which course [of] action is most appropriate. To do this, you will need to be able to decipher what is requi[red] of you, to develop the ability to ask questions, to look beneath the surface, and to develo[p a] deep understanding of what is needed. In short, you must become analytical. You will mo[ve] to a position of an analyst and problem solver – from where you will be able to ascert[ain] which rules are useful and assist in the delivery of care, and which do not. In so doing, y[ou] are preparing yourself to deliver effective care within modern healthcare services.

What is Analytical Thinking?

Initially, everyone will appear to know more than you, to be more skilled and more confide[nt.] As you gain experience, however, both in the classroom and in practice environmen[ts] it will be come clear that there is no one best or correct way of doing things and t[hat] different people will approach the same issue in a range of different ways. You will ne[ed] to be able to look at these different approaches in depth, to assess for yourself why so[me] approaches may work better than others, in some situations or for some patients. Y[ou] will need to learn to take nothing for granted – whether you are reading something i[n a] textbook (see Chapter 10 Critiquing the Healthcare Literature) or observing patient car[e in] a clinical environment.

There are the two key components of analytical thinking – 'looking at the detail' a[nd] 'taking nothing for granted'. There is nothing inherently difficult about either and by t[he] time we reach adulthood, we are experienced analytical thinkers. After all, most of us c[an] safely cross a busy road or manage a household budget simply by applying these t[wo] key components! Remember this when you are faced with an (apparently) challeng[ing] assignment or set of learning objectives.

Looking at the detail

To understand something we often need to simplify it. This is particularly important in the field of health care, where problems may be complex, where the root cause of ill-health may be masked by a range of different symptoms and where the desired outcome – a healthy nation – will only be achieved if we employ a wide range of different interventions and treatments.

Many assignments require some consideration of the need to simplify. You may be asked to *identify* the nutritional requirements of different age groups. The instruction to identify signals the first stage of an analytical process – that of demonstrating to your tutor or mentor that you have a simple understanding of human physiology and how needs differ with age. Instructions like 'identify', 'describe' and 'explain' test your basic knowledge and understanding.

Now that you have demonstrated that you can simplify a complex issue you will be asked to examine the detail of the component parts. *Analysis* is the second stage of examining the detail. You might be asked to analyse the factors contributing to the increased incidence of heart disease for a certain community or population group. Here you are asked to show that you understand that many factors – genetic, lifestyle, economic and social – may play a role and to demonstrate how these factors may interact with each other. Instructions like 'compare and contrast', 'discuss' or 'interpret' are all asking you to look at component parts and how they relate to one another.

Table 9.1 gives definitions of the most frequently used terms.

Taking nothing for granted

Once you have mastered the skill of dissecting your topic or challenge, you will move on to the more complex skill of judging the effectiveness of an idea or intervention and thinking through the consequences of a decision. This will require you to engage with the skills of *evaluation* and *structured reflection*.

When you are asked to *evaluate*, your tutor or mentor is testing your ability to measure and appraise – you may be asked which intervention may be most appropriate for a given patient? To answer adequately this kind of question you will need to have a yardstick or set of measurement criteria and to test out each intervention in terms of these criteria.

Table 9.1   Explanations of words used in analysis

What the task or assignment requires	What words will be used	What your tutor wants
Understanding (what is it that you need to comprehend)	Describe	Tell me the key features of an issue or problem
	Distinguish	Identify the differences between issues
	Identify	Select after consideration
	Explain	Make clear to someone
Analysis (can you break down the issue and examine the detail?)	Analyse	Break down into elements and explain how the elements together
	Categorize	Separate into clear divisions classes
	Compare and contrast	Set out the similarities and differences between
	Discuss	Produce a balanced argument
	Interpret	Translate into meaningful te…
Evaluation (can you judge and arrive at a decision?)	Evaluate/appraise	Judge the importance of particular interventions, models or theories
	Recommend	When you have made your judgement, advise anothe… on how to act
Reflect (can you stand back and, in a structured way, make sense of the experience you have had?)	Reflect	Make sense of your own role and responsibilities and in this way arrive at an understanding of what affects your performance

For example, when helping people to quit smoking our criteria might include fact… such as evidence of long-term effectiveness of the intervention, its acceptability to a… ease of use for the patient, the cost and availability of the intervention. Each possi… intervention – from cold-turkey, group or individual counselling, nicotine patches… hypnotherapy and so forth – could be tested against our criteria so as to assess and sel… the most appropriate treatment for our patient. Instructions such as 'appraise', 'advi… and 'recommend' all require this process of determining and measuring solutions agai… criteria so as to make an informed judgement.

The final level of analytical thinking requires you to integrate all that you have learnt so that you can gain personally from the experience and transfer this learning to new situations to solve new problems. Throughout your education you will be introduced to models of reflection to help you become a 'reflective practitioner'. These models will have one thing in common – they will help you to reflect in a structured way. From this you will become aware of your motivations and style of behaviour and will gain a better understanding of what affects your own performance. At a professional level, reflection will help to improve you judgement and decision-making ability; at a personal level it will help you to gain control of your emotions and responses in a clinical setting.

Developing Deep Approaches to Thinking and Learning

Asking questions

You may find it helpful to view thinking as a process of questioning so as to solve a puzzle or problem. We start with the simple questions such as 'what' 'where' 'when' and 'who', then dig below the surface to ask the question 'how' and end with a consideration of 'why'. When faced with a challenge – an assignment to write or the care of a patient – use the seven-step problem-solving framework below to help you identify appropriate questions.

1. **Define the problem**. Typical questions might include: What are the issues? What is the assessment asking me to do? What are the most significant aspects of the problem?
2. **Set priorities**. What is the most important issue I need to address first? What can I leave until later?
3. **Identify the possible causes of the problem**. What are the obvious symptoms of the problem? What is likely to be causing these? What do I know already? What guidance do I have?
4. **Collect and analyse relevant facts**. Where will I find the necessary information I need? Who will have had experience of working with this problem? How adequate/up-to-date is the information I have?
5. **Outline alternative courses of action**. What are my options?
6. **Evaluate the consequences of each course of action**. Which option seems best or most useful? What measurement criteria will be most useful? How do the alternative courses of action measure up against my evaluation criteria?
7. **Select and review**. Does the selected option work? If so why? If not, why not?

Looking below the surface

This process will take some time when you start to use it but, eventually, questioning v
become easier. The process will help you to look for some of the hidden meanings beh
problems, and to look below the surface to uncover less obvious causes and explanatio
It is important to work your way through to the 'why' questions. Only by doing this will y
get to the point where you challenge the surface or 'taken-for-granted' ways of workin

Our understanding of health and illness is not fixed or unchanging. Over time, n
information and better measurement tools enable us to generate new explanatio
models and theories. For example, with an increasing understanding of human psycholo
witchcraft explanations of atypical behaviour were replaced by mental health mod
Indeed, we must continue to develop a critical and analytical approach to our models a
theories and it is important to ask questions such as:

• Why is this regarded as the *best* explanation?
• What can it explain that other explanations can't?
• What can it not explain? And what might be the consequences of this?

Furthermore, in the United Kingdom, largely as a consequence of health policy and t
establishment of the National Health Service (NHS), our models of health have explor
and explained disease and illness. Only very recently have we considered explanations
well-being and good health. But by challenging the accepted way of thinking, we ha
started a radical process that will have a profound impact on your role as a nurse
midwife. No longer will you be expected to care only for the ill; now the promotion
healthy lifestyles will be at least as important.

This ability to think differently and to challenge all that is taken for granted lies at the he
of effective healthcare practice. However, thinking is not enough – the real evidence t
you have become analytical will lie in your behaviour.

Challenge without confrontation

The language of analysis can sound confrontational – after all, this entire chapter
about encouraging you to appraise, measure, evaluate and even dissect! Not langua
that we associate with productive and supportive relationships between people!
there is another hurdle that has to be overcome – the translation of analytical thinki
into appropriate behaviours. Once you have completed the analysis it might be wo
spending some time thinking through how you will present your argument. You mi

feel passionate about a particular approach, intervention or treatment but academic staff, when marking your essay, are more likely to be swayed by a balanced and reasoned argument. So marshal your evidence to support both sides of the argument and reach a conclusion based on a careful weighing up of the evidence (more of this in Chapter 10).

Similarly, senior staff or patients are not likely to respond well if their care or behaviour is challenged in a confrontational way. While you will be guided throughout your programme on how to navigate the difficult waters of interpersonal relationships and conflict management, you may find that the questioning strategies outlined above help.

Consider the way in which you pose a question. A question such as 'I wonder if you could tell me how effective this approach to care is in comparison with that one' is much less confrontational than 'why are you doing that?' Similarly, a perfectly innocent question can take on a new meaning by a rather blunt delivery. So, try to consider both your verbal and non-verbal behaviour.

Handling Ambiguity

Becoming analytical demands that you explore alternatives and make choices – you won't be able to avoid making decisions. Inevitably there will be times when, no matter how carefully you have planned or how meticulously you have followed the seven-step problem-solving framework above, you will still be unclear about the most appropriate option to select. At this point you *must* stop and ask advice from someone more experienced or better qualified than you are. You should then engage is some structured reflection – why were you not able to make the decision? What have you learnt that you will be able to apply to future situations and tasks? In this way you re-define step one of the problems solving framework (defining the problem) and engage with another cycle of analytical thinking and behaving.

Tips

- Becoming analytical is something that we learn – and like all learning requires practice and feedback on performance. Use every opportunity you have and pay attention to the feedback you receive
- Spend time thinking about the nature of the puzzle or problem you face. Plan and reflect before you jump in

- You have multiple sources of information to help you – texts, academic tutors, ment
  in practice, fellow students – use them all
- Remember
  - Look for the detail and take nothing for granted
  - Question and look below the surface
  - Develop behavioural strategies that help you to challenge what is taken for gran
    without seeming confrontational
  - You don't have to solve all problems – you do have to take advice and learn from t
    advice so that you can solve future problems.

Chapter 10

Critiquing the Healthcare Literature

by Steve Trenoweth and Simon Jones

In this chapter, you will:

- **Understand what is meant by critiquing the healthcare literature**
- **Appreciate why taking an informed, balanced and reasoned view of the literature is important in health care**
- **Be aware of what and how much to read**
- **Understand how you might manage, simplify and collate healthcare literature.**

Introduction

Being able to critique published healthcare literature is an important skill to develop
involves more than simply reading – it requires you to read and really think about w
you have read. It is not, therefore, something you can do passively – you have to be activ
engaged. And you have to think!

What do We Mean by Critiquing the Literature?

By critiquing the literature, we mean developing a questioning, analytical and reasor
approach to written material. The literature could be a research article in a journa
newspaper commentary, a chapter in a book, an editorial, a report, a set of guidelines
any other piece of writing in which someone is expressing their opinion. When you criti
written work, you should take an objective standpoint, highlighting both its merits and
limitations. In that way, when you come to make a final judgement on the quality of
work, your judgement is informed and based on a balanced interpretation of the facts
they are presented. The depth of critique will depend on: firstly, your knowledge of
subject area in question; secondly, your familiarity with the related published literatu
and thirdly, in the case of research, your understanding of the methods used.

While in this chapter we use the term 'critiquing the literature', the same process is oft
described in a variety of ways. For example, during your studies you may be askec
'critically review' or 'critically analyse' written materials. In either case the process that yo
be expected to go through will essentially be the same as the approach outlined here, t
is, one which is balanced and objective. The only difference being that we prefer the
of the word 'critique' as this implies a more balanced and objective approach to literat
evaluation. We have decided against the use of terms associated with the word 'critical
they tend to imply a negative approach to analysis.

Why Some People Find Critiquing Difficul

For various reasons some people find critiquing difficult. Sometimes people feel they
the necessary research knowledge and expertise. Sometimes people feel they don't kr
enough about the statistics and specialist jargon that are often used. Or they may just

that they don't yet have the 'right' to critique published work. Sometimes, people lack the confidence to critique; they feel that the author's opinions are more important than their own and believe that their own opinions would be of little interest to others. Consequently, those new to the process often tend to simply describe, or report, what the literature says rather than critiquing it.

To put this another way, there is a tendency for students new to critiquing to summarize or repeat what has been said by other people. However, it is important for you to embrace your own developing expertise and to realize that your views are extremely valid. You may not have read as much as the 'experts' but then they will not have the benefit of your particular and unique experience or perspective!

Why Critiquing is so Important in Health Care

You are embarking on a career in which you will be responsible for the health, safety and wellbeing of clients in your care. Central to this is being able to identify and meet the holistic needs of your clients and this is a complex process. You will be held accountable for your actions or omissions and it is essential, therefore, that you are able to justify any action that you take. This requires taking a professional and analytical stance to the care you offer your clients. It is essential, therefore, that in the pursuit of your chosen career, you undertake clinical decision making in an informed and balanced way and that you are able to justify the particular clinical path you have taken.

Adopting an analytical stance to your reading, then, is important not only for your studies, but the skills you learn through your active engagement with the literature will help you to become similarly analytical in your clinical practice. Here, you will almost certainly be faced with insufficient or contradictory information about the needs of people you will care for and you will almost certainly have to actively seek out information about your client. So, the skills you will learn in meeting the academic requirements of your course will also help you in responding to the needs of your clients.

It is a measure of our qualities and skills as healthcare practitioners that we are able to respond effectively to, and make sense of, the needs of those that rely on us for our help. This requires us to adopt a questioning, analytical, balanced and reasoned approach to issues. In this way, we will develop an understanding of the needs, wants and wishes of our clients and make a real difference to someone's life.

How Much and What to Read?

Some of the most frequent questions that our students ask are: How much do I need
read? How much is enough? What are the most important things that I should read? Her
our students are asking about the range and focus of their reading. We assume that o
students mean 'how should I target my reading?' rather than 'what is the minimum readir
I need to do?'

It is difficult to provide rules here but there are a number of issues that you will need
bear in mind. Firstly, it usually follows that the more you read the greater your grasp of a
issue will be. That is, when you become exposed to more ideas, the greater your grasp
that topic will be. You become aware of the various theories and facets of that topic, ar
this can give you a clearer picture about how much is known – and how much is not y
known! It is useful to get literature which seems contradictory, or at least gives you bo
sides of an argument. This will, in turn, allow you to approach the literature in a muc
more balanced and analytical way. Of course, there is an upper limit to how much you ca
reasonably be expected to read. Often this will depend on the amount of time availab
to you given the assessment submission date and other demands in you life. Howeve
with effective time management it is possible to balance the demands of home and yo
programme.

Try to find the *most important* literature first. Here, it is essential that you attend all lectur
and we would strongly recommend that you pay close attention, as this will often not on
help you to grasp a particular issue but often direct you to some of the most significa
literature, which you should then try to follow up. This is a very useful starting point. Als
we would advise you to consult your programme documentation for recommended
essential reading lists. The lists are carefully thought out by academic staff to help yc
navigate your way through the healthcare literature. Of course, you may wish to see
additional and specific guidance and the personal recommendations of essential readir
materials from your personal tutor, other lecturers and/or clinical staff.

Also, we would recommend that you try to obtain literature that brings you up to date wit
what is known at the present time about an issue. Here, recommended course textbool
can be a great introduction. Indeed, there are some superb books that can simplify issue
and point you in the right direction. We suggest that you purchase at least one of these – be
try before you buy! If your library has a good range of the textbooks recommended f
your programme, take a few out on loan to see which one(s) seem most helpful for you.

You must be aware, though, that textbooks contain mostly secondary sources of information in that they often give only a brief overview or summary of what may be a very large body of literature on a given subject. Sometimes, a textbook can give a particular slant to healthcare issues based on the author's own interpretation or bias. Here, we would recommend that you try to seek out, as much as possible, the primary or original sources of information and come to your own conclusions.

There are other potential problems with relying solely on textbooks for your information. It is important to be aware that our knowledge about health issues develops all the time and this is why when we use literature, either to help us complete a theoretical assignment or to provide effective health care, we must use information that is current and up to date. Due to the time it takes to produce textbooks, sometimes a year or two or even more, they cannot hope to keep up with the most recent developments.

You will often hear reference made to best available evidence. By this, people are referring to research and the opinions of experts which identify what is thought to be the most effective way of providing health care. In trying to find this evidence, we would recommend that in the first instance you visit the website of the National Institute for Health and Clinical Excellence (NICE), whose guidance is based on large and thorough systematic reviews (these being an extensive review and analysis of previously published research literature on a given healthcare issue). Increasingly, you will find other systematic and general literature reviews in the nursing, midwifery and medical literature.

Additionally, it is absolutely vital for modern healthcare practitioners to consider and act upon the views of their patients/clients. Here, there are many reports and general guidance made by user groups (as well as articles and book chapters written by patients/clients) which can help to provide care that is not only effective but also sensitive to the diverse and complex needs of your client group.

This brings us to another very important point. Health care exists within a political context. It is vital that you are aware of the policies that have been instigated by Government which will help you to establish the legal and political framework within which health care takes place.

Finally, be aware that even the best available evidence may not help us to respond to some of the more complex issues. There are often ethical dilemmas which healthcare practitioners face, and here you will often find yourself referring to the guidance and standards issued by the Nursing and Midwifery Council (NMC) in order to help you judge the ethical merits of a particular argument or article.

When I'm Reading, What Should I Look Out For?

Although you should always take an objective standpoint when critiquing the work others, there is also a place in every critique for issues that relate to your own person reflection. This is how you are able to make a personal connection to your literature critiq and begin to develop your own ideas as a researcher.

In Table 10.1 we suggest some of the most important issues to be aware of when you a critiquing the healthcare literature. Below we highlight some of the key issues and expla why we think they are important.

What is the *best* type of literature?

There are many forms that healthcare literature can take – from traditional quantitati research (such as study of a healthcare intervention which reliably demonstrates improved clinical outcome for a particular disease) to research which is more qualitati in nature (e.g. which might be an observational study or an investigation into how peop cope with and experience a particular illness). Sometimes, you will find an account

Table 10.1   Checklist – What should I look out for when critiquing the literature?

- What type of literature is it? (e.g. research article, editorial, etc.)
- Does it constitute 'best available evidence'?
- When was it written? Is it relevant? Is it still relevant?
- In which country was it published?
- Who is the author? If it is a piece of research, who funded the study?
- Are conclusions justified? Have the authors jumped to conclusions without sufficiently arguin their case or providing sufficient evidence? Have they considered the limitations of their research?
- Do you understand it? Is it clear?
- Does the work remind you of a care scenario you have been involved in? Does it help you to understand that scenario or healthcare issues? Does it seem relevant to that care scenario? Does the work seem relevant to your experience?
- Do you agree with the inferences and conclusions? If so, why? If not, why not? Does the work remind you of a care scenario you have been involved in?
- If there is contradictory evidence, which argument do you find more persuasive ? Why? Are there more supporters of one side of an argument than the other?
- Does the work have something important to say about health care? What are the implications for your chosen profession?
- Can you think of ways that the study could have been improved? How would you have done it

someone's opinion or a vivid account of a personal experience of illness. Much of this literature will be of use to you in your studies, and will be of value in assisting you to become reflective, professional practitioners capable of delivering effective nursing care.

But which is the best? This is a very difficult question to answer! Great emphasis is placed today on the use of research studies, particularly those that seek to provide evidence of the effectiveness of a particular healthcare intervention over another – that is, best available evidence. This is, of course, very important information and if you are looking to recommend a particular healthcare intervention which is most likely to work, you should look for studies that are 'randomized controlled trials' or systematic reviews, such as those available at NICE. Also, be aware of the social policy context or any good practice guides that have been issued by the Department of Health.

However, you must not overlook work in which people are expressing their personal opinions (particularly if these people are well known or an expert in their field). It is also vital to understand the experiences of those who receive our nursing care and thus the written descriptions of experiences of patients/clients can provide a vital insight and help you develop empathy. It is not enough to provide effective care if it is not acceptable to your clients. That is, you must not blindly recommend best evidence without considering the importance of seeking your client's permission. Remember modern health care is something that we do *with* our patients and not *to* them, and this must be reflected in your critique and indeed in your clinical practice. But at the same time be careful that you do not generalize from one client's written experience and assume that this is the same for all.

Where to find the literature?

There are a few issues here that you need to be mindful of. It is not wise to simply consult the textbooks. This predominantly comprises secondary sources of information – that is, the author's secondhand account of research and other literature. Textbooks can only condense information and give you a brief overview of major findings. Crucially, in terms of critiquing, they can be viewed as a tour guide that draws your attention to what they believe to be the most important points of interest. Sometimes they might miss out crucial facts which might have been of relevance to you, that you could have found if you had taken the time to explore the primary sources (that is, the original research articles, published mostly in journals). Many journals have a very rigorous review process, which means that work submitted by authors/researchers (including statistical analyses) has to be reviewed by people who have expertise in the article's field of study before it is published.

If the work does not meet the journal's strict standards of quality it will be rejected. This your quality assurance that the information contained in such articles is sound.

Be very careful about relying on information available on websites. While there a some important websites you should consult regularly – the NMC (www.nmc-uk.or NICE (www.nice.org.uk) and Department of Health (www.dh.gov.uk) are obvic examples – some of the information posted online can lack credibility and may n constitute best available evidence. Information may be politically or personally motivate may be inaccurate and may reflect the sometimes very narrow (or indeed biased) vie of the website authors. Instead, try as much as possible to come to your own conclusic by seeking out primary sources of information, available from journals either online (health databases and search engines) or libraries (please see chapter 8).

Which country was it written in/does it apply to?

In your critique, it is important to consider the national context. That is, we must careful that we do not simply apply evidence found in another country to the Unit Kingdom context without qualification (and of course vice versa). There might well differences in terms of cultural expectations and views, health policies, resources or the ve healthcare system itself might have implications for the transferability and the relevar of findings.

When was it written?

Our students often ask questions such as, 'this work was published in 1987, can I still u it?' It is difficult to give answers to questions concerning the validity of published we in relation to when it was published, but you must ask yourself – is the work releva today? There are many studies that we could cite that seemingly appear outdated t are (arguably) still relevant today – for example, Zubin and Spring (1977), Carper (197 Indeed, in this book you will find references made to work by Benner (1984), who mal important points that have resonance today. However, some aspects of governmer healthcare policies from previous administrations are not relevant today or have be superseded by others.

Information obtained from textbooks can often be out of date. Whenever you can y must try to obtain the latest edition of textbooks. Also, be aware of the difference betwe the publication date and the reprint date. The actual date of the work is the copyrigh publication date.

The rule of thumb is to keep up to date with what is current, but it is important not to dismiss research or other literature simply because of its age. You must make an informed decision.

What is the author's motivation?

You must be aware that there are some factors that might have a bearing on their author's interpretation of their findings. Some journals now require authors or researchers to declare their interests. For example, if you were undertaking research into wound care that had been commissioned and funded by a company that manufactured medical dressings, which your study subsequently recommended, you could be accused of bias. Sometimes, authors might be trying to make (party) political points or influence a political agenda, and remember while your critique should take into account different voices, you should take a balanced view of such things.

How to Manage, Simplify and Sort Through Literature

Ok, so you searched the literature on an online database, such as MEDLINE (see Chapter 8) and you've found over 100 references to articles that all appear to be relevant to you. But what now? Well, you have two options. Option 1, you spend weeks, even months, tracking down and reading every single one of those articles from beginning to end. Or Option 2, you take a more considered, systematic approach to your reading. Of course you are free to choose Option 1, which unfortunately many students do, but we strongly recommend that you instead choose Option 2 and suggest you do so using the following steps:

Step 1 Make a list of all the questions that you are hoping to answer. It is important that you are clear what these are as they will help you to focus your search and allow you to decide which documents you'll need to retrieve for critique. If you find it difficult to think of questions, it may help you to think about exactly why you are searching the literature and what you are trying to find out.

Step 2 Run your literature search, making sure to print off, or make a note of, the title and abstract information for every reference that comes up in your search.

Step 3 For each reference you need to decide whether or not to retrieve and critique the related full-text document. To make this decision, read through the title and abstract of each reference, asking yourself the following two questions:

- Would this document answer any of my questions? (see Step 1)
- Would this document enhance my knowledge and understanding, in some w of the subject I'm concerned with?

If the answer is 'yes' to either of these questions then the reference should marked for inclusion in your critique and a copy of the related full-text docum should be retrieved. However, if the answer is 'no' to both of these questie then you should disregard that reference and not worry about retrieving full-text document it relates to. There is no point in spending hours tracking do and reading documents that clearly have nothing to do with the issues you interested in. However, if after reading through a reference's title and abstract still have any doubts at all as to whether the related full-text document would of any use to you, then you should retrieve it and read through the main bod that document before deciding whether it should be included in or excluded fr your critique. Do not be surprised if only a minority of the references that came in your literature search are included in your critique.

Step 4 You should now have a stack of documents, each of which you feel will to your understanding of your chosen topic. Your aim now is to read eacl these documents thoroughly, systematically summarizing that content whic important to you. The easiest way to do this is to carefully read each document us a fluorescent pen to highlight relevant information such as the title, the autho the aims/objectives, methods, findings, conclusions and recommendations. M sure you have a good quality research dictionary close to hand and look up words you don't understand. You may have to read some documents several tii to make sure you have highlighted everything you feel is relevant to your topic. N use what you have highlighted to write a short summary of the document – mal sure to note your thoughts on its strengths, weaknesses and any ways in which study could have been improved.

Step 5 You can now use each summary to form the basis of your critique of each docum Using the summary will help focus your critique only on that information wl is important to you. Remember to remain balanced and objective at all times apply what you have learnt from this chapter to form what should be a though analytical judgement of both the merits and limitations of the document.

Look for the Gaps

When you are reading, you must consider not only what the literature is saying, but what it doesn't say. You might have noticed an important gap in our knowledge understanding of a particular issue and in your critique you should highlight this. You might also have formed an idea about what you think is relevant to a particular healthcare issue that no one seems to have considered. This is often the springboard for the start of a new piece of research and a good indication that your skills of critiquing have led you to think in new, innovative and creative ways.

Tips

To succeed in critiquing the healthcare literature:

* Try not to merely report or describe – develop a questioning, analytical and reasoned approach to written material
* Plan your work well ahead of the submission date, as this will give you time to obtain necessary information and think about, and reflect upon, healthcare issues
* Read widely – the more you read the greater your grasp of an issue will be
* Do not rely solely on textbooks – try to obtain primary sources of information wherever possible
* Try not to rely on information obtained from the Internet, unless the websites are reputable
* Ensure that you have access to, and regularly use good healthcare search engines.

References

Benner, P. (1984) *From Novice to Expert: Excellence and Power in Clinical Nursing Practice.* Menlo Park, Addison-Wesley.

Carper, B.A. (1978) Fundamental patterns of knowing in nursing, *Advances in Nursing Science*, **1**, 13–23.

Zubin, J. and Spring B. (1977) Vulnerability – a new view of schizophrenia. *Journal of Abnormal Psychology*, **86**(2), 103–24.

Chapter 11

Organizing and Planning Your Theoretical Assessments

by Steve Trenoweth

In this chapter you will develop an understanding of:

- **How best to organize your time**
- **How to adopt an organized approach to your theoretical assessments**
- **Strategies to develop, structure and organize your work**
- **The importance of organizing articles and other literature.**

Importance of Organizing Your Time

Organizing your theoretical assessments is a part of a much wider issue – that of organizi
yourself! While it is important to maintain a focus to your studies, it is also vital that y
maintain an appropriate work/life balance. By this I mean that you are able to satisfactor
manage the competing demands on your life while you are studying (i.e. in meeting t
programme requirements but not at the expense of sacrificing your relationships w
your friends, family and significant others).

I am fully aware that, in the real world, many students might have to financially supp
themselves, their children and their families by working bank or agency nursing shifts
other part-time work. Unfortunately, in my experience, students have sometimes plac
their programme in jeopardy by prioritizing this extracurricular working.

Nursing and midwifery programmes are personally and intellectually challenging a
can be a considerable drain on your time. Sometimes, it is clear that students ha
underestimated how long it will take them to complete a particular theoretical assessme
They have 'left it to the last minute' and here work submitted often has a rushed feel, w
poor attention to detail and can be very poorly organized.

So, in order to succeed in your studies, you will need to adopt a disciplined and balanc
approach to yourself and your studies. In this chapter, I focus on assisting you to add
an organized and systematic approach in the planning of your academic course work a
essays, and to offer a framework to help you, and your ideas, to shine!

General Advice

Here, I offer you in broad terms some advice on organizing an academic essay. It is essent
though that you follow any specific advice, guidance or requirements given to you on yo
particular programme.

Firstly, give yourself sufficient time to get yourself organized! You are likely to encoun
difficulties if you leave planning or writing your essay until the last minute. While the ess
may seem quite straightforward at first glance, you might well find that when you start
consider this in more depth that it has quite complex clinical and professional implicatio
If you know that you have to hand in an essay in eight weeks' time start your preparatic
now! It is also important to remember that the submission date for any theoretical work

not the date it is due in, but the *last* date it is due in! I strongly advise you to hand your work in a day or two before the submission date – I have encountered students who experience last minute problems with handing in their essays (in the form of travel difficulties, computer or printer problems, etc.). Not only does this unnecessarily and dramatically increase your stress levels, but there is often an academic penalty for late submissions!

You must also be mindful of the word limit of your assignment or essay. Most universities have a penalty if you stray too far over this limit – sometimes this can be as much as a 10% reduction of your overall mark! Furthermore, if your work is under this word limit, there may not be an academic penalty as such, but it is unlikely that you will have fully explored the issues and your work may be accused of lacking depth and detail. So, an essential element of being organized is aiming, as closely as is possible, for the required word limit. This can be quite an academic challenge as it requires you to be focused on the assignment requirements and to try to avoid bringing in irrelevant information.

Planning Your Work

I cannot stress the importance of this enough – before you start to write up your essay or other theoretical course work, plan it! Developing a structured plan is an essential academic skill that will help you to help you organize your ideas and will provide an important framework for your essay or other academic work. Furthermore, a good plan gives you (and a tutor with whom you may wish to discuss this) a clear overview of how you will address the essay requirements. It also helps you to see which of your ideas are connected, thereby increasing narrative flow. So, you should take some time to develop your ideas; to structure and organize your thoughts so that they can be presented in a comprehensive and coherent way.

Now, imagine if you had been set this assignment.

Consider the following statement:

People's psychological response to a physical illness might be overlooked by healthcare practitioners and this is likely to hinder the delivery of effective holistic care.

Do you feel this statement is justified? How might nurses/midwives provide effective holistic care to their patients?

How might you approach this? Where would you start? Before you write anything, make sure you fully understand what is required of you in the assignment. You will certainly need to give this some thought particularly if you have not encountered some of the concepts before. At first, it may not be completely clear what is expected, or you might have a limited understanding of the issues. My advice is, before you make your plan, read around the subject area. This is where textbooks can be a real help in giving you a broad overview. You could also search databases for literature reviews or good practice guidelines. You might also like to discuss this further with your personal tutor or have a chat to a student colleague. However you wish to proceed it is wise to have a general understanding of the issues before planning your work.

Strategies to Develop, Structure and Organize Your Work

There are many methods which can help you to do this and I mention two here – the Highlight Key Words method and the Spider Diagrams method.

Highlight key words method

Let's return to the above assignment that you have just been set. Which issues seem most important to you here? I have highlighted those issues that I feel are most important.

> Consider the following statement:
>
> People's <u>psychological response</u> to a physical illness might be <u>overlooked</u> by healthcare practitioners and is likely to hinder their delivery of <u>effective holistic care</u>.
>
> Do you feel this statement is justified? How might nurses/midwives provide effective holistic care to their patients?

Once you have highlighted key words, you might wish to search a health literature database to clarify issues. For example, what exactly is effective care? Or holistic care for that matter? Is there any evidence at all that nurses/midwives do overlook the psychological needs of their clients?

Once you have researched the area, you will feel ready to write your plan – that is, structure your ideas and thoughts so as to present them in a way that is sensible to another reader. I suggest that you write each highlighted key word at the top of separate pages of A4 paper – this allows you the opportunity to brainstorm your ideas and the space to annotate (i.e. make comments) on them. You might also want to make specific reference to issues that seemed interesting or important to you or particular articles or theories that seem particularly relevant. Use bullet points – this allows each idea or note to yourself to stand out clearly, but do leave space around them to add further comments.

For example:

'Psychological Response'

- How people might feel, think or see their problem
- This might influence how people behave
- Feelings of sadness, hopelessness, anger at having a physical illness have been reported
- People can have mental health problems resulting from their physical health problems. This can have a significant effect on their recovery and clinical outcomes
- How do mental health nurses and other mental health professionals respond to their client's psychological needs?

'Overlooked'

- Is there any evidence for this?
- As an adult nurse, would I be able to respond to psychological needs?
- If I were to overlook people's psychological responses to their illness, why might this be? For example, there might be limited time to meet psychological needs, and if I didn't have training in counselling techniques how might I do this?

'Effective Holistic Care'

- What is holistic care? Seems to encompass various needs: biological/physical, social, psychological, spiritual
- What is effective holistic care? Give examples of physical care which has a psychological component, for example cardiac rehabilitation programmes. I must remember to look at research evidence for other examples, for example systematic reviews, good practice guidelines, user's experiences
- How do we know it is effective? Evaluating our clinical interventions, measuring clinical outcomes
- How might we provide holistic care? What might work? How do I know this?

This method is useful to help you to think things through. It also helps you to structu your work – particularly if you think of each page as a section or a number of paragrap around a theme. It is a very neat and ordered way of planning your work which may s people who like to approach their work in a logical, linear and very structured way.

Spider diagrams method

Another helpful way of organizing your work (and one that I use and recommend our students all the time) is the so-called spider diagrams method. (Those suffering fr arachnophobia should be aware that this doesn't actually involve you having any cont with spiders!)

This approach is logical but is much more 'messy' than the linear 'key words' method can be invaluable to help you link ideas together in a coherent fashion. Here, I take y through how you might like to develop your own spider diagrams. There are many w. of doing this, but I find this way helps (you can combine it with the highlight key wo method if it helps).

Look at your assignment again.

Consider the following statement:

People's psychological response to a physical illness might be overlooked by healthcare practitioners and is likely to hinder their delivery of effective holistic care.

Do you feel this statement is justified? How might nurses/midwives provide effective holistic care to their patients?

In the first instance, consider what this assignment is actually asking you to write abc What is the most important theme or issue? Here, you will certainly need to th this through. You might have to look at the literature or perhaps have a chat to y personal tutor. On reflection, we think the focus of this essay is on the preparednes: nurses/midwives to provide effective holistic care – this becomes the body of your 'spi' (Figure 11.1). I suggest you write this in the centre of a piece of paper.

Then, ask yourself what sub-themes or issues are related to this that you will need consider? Well, some of these have already been suggested to you in the assignm guidelines. You might have highlighted key words. In our example, certainly, you need to consider what is meant by *holistic care* and also how that care might be *effec*

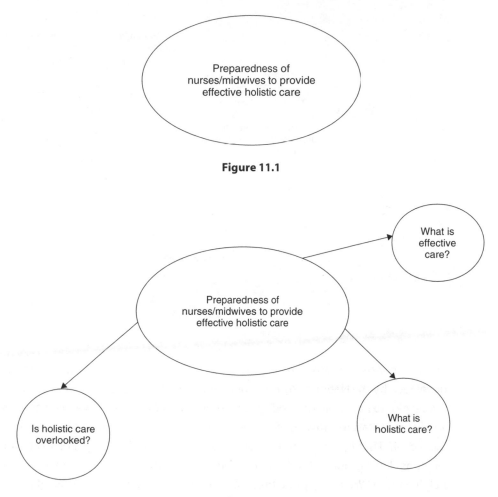

Figure 11.1

Figure 11.2

(and indeed how we would know this). We will also need to explore the possibility that nurses/midwives have *overlooked* psychological care and you are asked to give your opinion here. These ideas are linked to the spider's body by 'legs' (Figure 11.2).

Now let's take one of these 'legs'. What do we mean by *effective care*? How would we know if our care works? Simply, *what* is effective care? Let's brainstorm this. (Again, if you feel unsure about any of these terms or are not clear about how to proceed, then take some time out to research the area before planning.)

If we were looking to clarify what we meant by effective care, we would certainly need to consult the literature. But what sort of literature? General evidence of effectiveness of

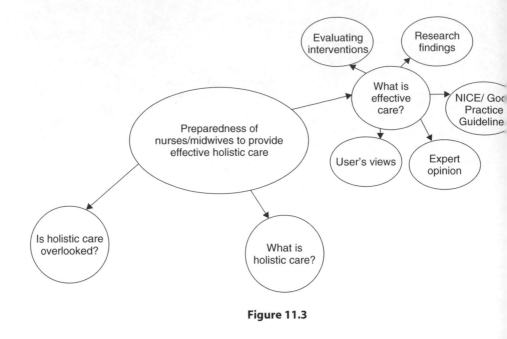

Figure 11.3

healthcare interventions can come from research, systematic reviews, clinical guideli[n]
developed by the National Institute for Health and Clinical Excellence (NICE), good prac[tice]
guidelines, expert opinion, and user's experiences. But even if we were to provide [care]
which the literature shows is effective, how would we know if it was working for a spe[cific]
individual? That is, we need to evaluate our own clinical interventions with a partic[ular]
client or client group – that is, do our patients feel that the care that we offer is actu[ally]
helping them? We can capture these ideas by adding this to our diagram (Figure 11.3)

Now, we can even take this a step further! When we look back at the assignm[ent]
requirements, you are asked how nurses/midwives might provide effective holistic car[e to]
their patients. So, let's think about *how* we might evaluate our interventions. On our sp[ider]
diagram we feel that this related to effective care. Clearly, when we need to evaluate [the]
effectiveness of our care, we need to consider if the person is personally experiencing [an]
abatement of, or relief from, their symptoms. That is, we must try to capture the clie[nt's]
views (via *self-report*) as to how well they believe healthcare interventions are working [for]
them. We could ascertain this not only by taking appropriate *physical measurements* [(e.g.]
temperature, blood pressure, bedsore, etc.) or by using objective and appropriate *scale[s/]
tools*. We can add this to our diagram (Figure 11.4).

If we were to continue, a more detailed spider diagram may look like Figure 11.5.

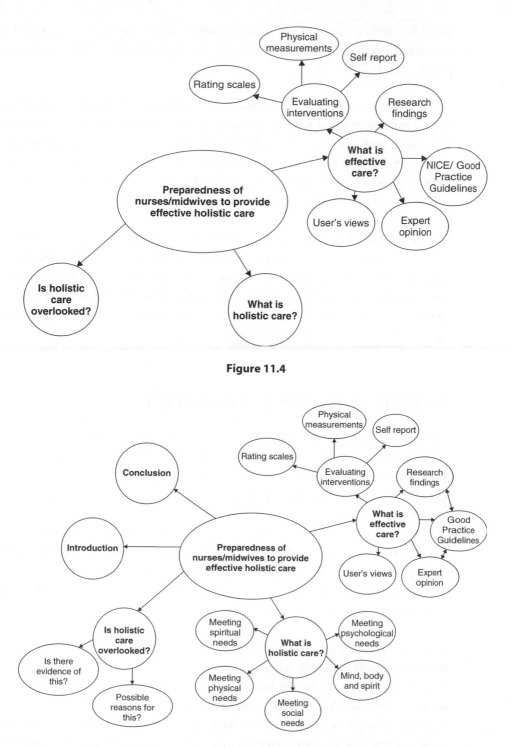

Figure 11.4

Figure 11.5

When you look at Figure 11.5, it is easy to retrace your steps and see how your ideas
connected. You might have your own ideas about what to add and take away. How mi
you develop this further?

I have added an Introduction and Conclusion bubble just to remind you to include the
As you can see, the end product is a very detailed, organized and well integrated p
and, reassuringly if you are an 'arachnophobe', in no way resembles a spider! It is easy
add or remove further ideas or move things around in a way that makes sense to you
helps you give a coherent answer to the question. You might also want to add support
references or research articles to illustrate or support points you raise.

In reality, it is unlikely that you will ever have a fully completed spider diagram – ev
time you return to it you are likely to want to make changes based on not only h
your own ideas about the issue changes, but also reflective of development in
understanding about an issue (as reported in the research literature) and changes wit
healthcare provision. Try not to worry about this – and remember that your essay sho
be a reflection of the best you can do at any given time.

Organizing Your Research

If you research your essays well, you will soon find that you have quite a collection
research papers and journal articles. It is also always worth keeping your essay plans saf
you may need to make reference to them again in the future. The message is simple – ne
throw anything away! An essential academic discipline is the ability to organize referen
so that you may be able to return to them at some point in the future. It is amazing h
often you will return to some of these articles so try to get into the habit of systematic
filing your references often. However, I am not suggesting that you develop a catalogu
system like you would find in a library! Just a few box files clearly labelled (e.g. with ti
such as Diabetes, Autism, Health Promotion, etc.) can assist you to quickly find tha
important article should you need it again in the future – and chances are that you wil

If you are confident in using Information Technology, you may like to start an electro
library for your 'downloads'. Many of the online health databases (such as MEDLINE, O
CINAHL, etc.) have the facility for you to save references electronically, albeit for y
personal use only. (You must be aware that copyright law applies to electronic copie
references and you must not share such files.) Create a folder system (imagine them to
electronic box files) for your references – and when you save them make sure that you

them a file name which is meaningful to you. Be aware, that if you are using Adobe Acrobat, the reference is most likely to have a numerical file name, such as '0009–654–3425'. If you save using this file name, you are unlikely to remember what it is referring to and if you have saved a number of files like this, you are going to have to spend a lot of time opening them all to find the one you want! (This is a mistake I have made in the past!) So when you are saving highlight the filename, delete it and type in a name that is more meaningful to you and that more adequately reflects the content of the article you are saving.

Working with Others

Finally, a few words of advice about working with others, as this can have implications for you all when you organize your work. The university may expect you to collaborate in the development of a group project and this can pose additional problems in terms of your combined work if it is not well organized. I would advise that you plan your group work thoroughly and that everyone clearly understands, and can account for, their individual responsibilities to the group.

You may also be asked to work collaboratively and submit an individual assignment. A good example of this might be a group of students who undertake a field study of voluntary health services within a given community. As a group you will most likely identify similar health related statistics and other information (e.g. birth rates, mortality rates, incidence of particular diseases, etc.). However, while you may share the same or similar factual information, it should be clear what your individual interpretation and contribution is to the overall completed work.

Tips

- Allow yourself time to complete theoretical assignments
- Try to adopt an organized approach to your studies
- Plan your assignments – if you are unclear what the assignment is asking you to do, then spend some time reading around the subject or discuss this with your tutor
- Catalogue and store your references safely.

Chapter 12

How to Write in an Academic Way

by Julia Magill-Cuerden

This chapter considers:

- **The importance of presenting your theoretical work in an academic way**
- **What you might consider when developing the text**
- **Areas to consider in developing your writing style.**

Introduction

Throughout your programme, you will be required to complete written assignmer Though these assignments may take different forms, developing your writing style in way that is accepted for academic work is crucial to your final success. Learning how develop your knowledge and skills in the form of writing is as important as other parts your education during your programme.

The majority of writing that you will undertake will need to be written factually. T means that when you write you often need to refer to knowledge or evidence within t professional or public domain, which you must reference consistently and accurately.

In general, if you are writing an academic essay you should not make unfound assumptions based on your own personal beliefs – unless, of course, you are writing explicitly reflective piece. That is, when writing reflectively, you will often be required refer back to your own personal experiences such as those arising from working w patients/clients, and to consider your own personal feelings and any issues which ha implications for your personal and professional growth.

When writing academically you will often need to find a style of writing that argues differe points within the text. This means that you will need to discuss ideas relating to an iss from different sources or authors, ensuring that you represent their views accurately. Y will then often need to compare and contrast the various (and sometimes contradicto views, drawing them together before coming to some form of conclusion on the issue yourself, justifying your argument based on what you have read and often what you ha experienced in clinical practice.

Getting Started

Getting started on writing an assignment can sometimes be very difficult. You might w encounter writers' block, or be unsure as to how to approach the issue you are requil to analyse (Chapter 9 might be helpful here as its gives you some tips on becomi analytical). Don't worry, though, if you have problems starting – this is perfectly norm Often people encounter problems at the outset because they have not planned th work sufficiently beforehand and therefore I would strongly advise that before you be writing, as suggested in the previous chapter, you plan your work.

In this chapter, we are considering how you might express yourself once you have developed the plan for your work and are in the process of writing it up. People approach writing in many different ways. You may write 'serially', that is, you might write different sections of your work at a time and then put each piece together to complete the work – like a quilt! For example, if you are writing about different cultural beliefs of health and illness, you may wish to have a section on how different cultures perceive the aetiology of illness; another on how such beliefs affect the treatment and care; and perhaps another on how we respect cultural differences in our clinical practice. The important task here is to ensure that there is a clear link between these sections, otherwise it may feel disjointed and lack a good narrative flow.

Alternatively, you may write 'holistically'. Writers who develop their work this way may write the complete text and then produce a number of drafts until they are satisfied that the work conveys what they mean to say. This can be very time consuming, however, and requires you to have a very good focus on all the various ideas and issues in your work.

There is no right or wrong way here – it is really what you feel most comfortable with. I would suggest that whatever approach you take you write a section of your work that you feel most knowledgeable about first. This will help you to 'break the ice' and give you that all important confidence to get started.

Presentation of Your Ideas

When you are writing, you are conveying your ideas to a person who does not know the steps you have taken in your thinking about the topic. Therefore, you will need to think how you may convey simply to others your views about the issue and how you have come to your conclusions. If I were to say to you that I believe the moon were made of cheese, I'm sure you would like to know how I came to such a conclusion and where I obtained my evidence! It may help to break down some ideas you have into several simple steps and then write about each one in a logical and sequential process. This will also help you to develop a clear and sound rationale to underpin your argument or conclusions.

Your written text should appear in an ordered and logical sequence so the reader can see how you have undertaken the working out of your ideas. That is, you should present your ideas so that they build to a clear conclusion. This may be similar to the way in which you may have undertaken a mathematical problem where you show the individual stages of the sum to illustrate how you came to the result.

Like any good story, all academic essays require a beginning, a middle and an end. At the outset of your assignment, you will need to clearly introduce your work. This will set the tone of your work and offer an overview of the purpose of your essay. That is, you will need to state, succinctly and accurately, what you are going to talk about in your essay. This may be a summary of your essay plan. It is difficult to give hard and fast rules here about how long the introduction should be, but (unless you have been given instructions otherwise) your introduction should take up no more that about 10% of the overall word count.

In the main body of your essay, you will need to expand on the issues you have promised to talk about in your introduction. Always have your plan to hand when writing the main body – this will help you keep on track and remain organized. Remember, if you have said in your introduction that you will write about something, make sure that you do!

Your conclusion should obviously be related to the introduction and the main body of your essay. Here, do not bring in new information, data or research. The point of a conclusion is to succinctly summarize and clearly draw together the most important points you have explored in the main body. This gives you the opportunity to reinforce the most important points you wish the marker to be aware of.

Considerations When Developing the Text

In this section, I will take you through some of the issues that I would advise you to consider when presenting your work, as this can assist greatly in conveying your ideas. However, you will need to consider the guidelines you have been given by your university. It is important to note here that each university will have its own specific expectations about how to present academic assignments, and I would advise you in the first instance to seek these out.

Writing objectively

The challenge is to write as objectively as you can. Try to avoid the use of adverbs (words which modify a verb, such as quickly, patiently) and adjectives (words which describe nouns, such as small, yellow) if they do not present factual information. Adverbs and adjectives can reflect your own personal views or opinions. For example, 'he was an old Asian man'. What do we mean by old? How old is old? What do we mean by Asian? Now you may know what you mean – but this may be completely different from other people's interpretation. Use instead a specific sentence, such as, 'he was a 70-year-old man born in India'.

Conversational versus academic writing

Previously, your writing may have been in a style that is similar to the language that you use in conversations. This can be quite informal, and sometimes can include colloquial expressions. Sometimes, such writing can be quite descriptive as it might narrate particular events in your life, for example in letter writing or if you are compiling a journal or diary.

Sometimes, in your programme you may be asked to write a case study or a personal reflective account, and under these circumstances you can write more descriptively and conversationally.

When writing for academic purposes, it is usual to adopt a more formal written style, where you will often need to identify, discuss or critique professional knowledge. This kind of writing requires you to be analytical and critical of the issues that you are presenting and to demonstrate new information that you have gained from it. Thus, you are attempting to draw upon information and justify your position. Such style of writing can seem more formal and impersonal.

Try to avoid asking questions in your text but rather put your question as an issue which you will then discuss. For example, instead of asking 'So why should the patient get up and be mobile soon after an operation?' turn this around into a statement, such as 'Early mobilization and ambulation of a patient after an operation is advised to reduce the possibility of deep vein thrombosis following surgery and it will also assist in reducing pain thresholds'. This latter sentence gives the reader factual information showing your understanding of the issues.

Personal and impersonal styles of writing

There is a debate about whether student nurses or midwives should write in an impersonal or personal tone in academic essays. In an impersonal style of writing there is no reference made to you as the writer. For example:

> ... the nurse–patient relationship is not a uniform professionalized blueprint but rather a kaleidoscope of intimacy and distance in some of the most dramatic, poignant, and mundane moments of life. (Benner 1984, xxii)

Thus, in impersonal styles, you write without reference to yourself, or your feelings or ideas.

However, there may be occasions when it is appropriate for you to write in the personal voice, such as when writing a personal reflective piece. Here, it is often appropriate to use the personal pronouns (such as 'I' or 'we') especially where a personal interpretation of issue or a clinical event is required. For example:

> I am distressed when nurses rigidly follow doctor's orders for diet or other comfort measure. when the order is clearly outdated and the patient's comfort is sacrificed to a ritualized chair of command. (Benner 1984, 144)

So, it is important to consider the tone of your written work and when it is appropriate use the personal or impersonal voice. Remember that you can express the same idea different ways, for example:

> I believe it is important to consider cultural needs when undertaking a comprehensive nursing assessment. (Personal)
>
> It is important to consider cultural needs when undertaking a comprehensive nursing assessment. (Impersonal)

Narrative flow

When you think of your written work, try to plan it so that it appears as if you are writing a story. For example, when discussing a problem you may wish to consider the aetiology and clinical symptoms of an illness, and then progress to exploring the different possible ways of treating and caring for the problem before reaching a conclusion. While there may be different ways of arranging your ideas, carefully consider the links between themes that emerge from your reading. It is important that you develop your ideas in a logical way that will assist with the narrative flow of the your work.

Think about your favourite novel. It is likely to have a number of important ingredients:

- It is likely to be a story which makes sense to you
- The plot or story will be interesting and pleasurable read
- It will be written in a tone and style which is understandable to you
- The characters 'speak' to you
- It has a good narrative flow and is easy to follow
- There will be no erratic punctuation, no spelling mistakes or grammatical errors which might detract you from the story
- It might even make you think!

In short, it is most likely that your favourite novel will make sense to you because it presented well and is well organized. These are central features that you should try capture when you are presenting your essays or other written programme materials.

It is important to remember that when you are writing an essay, or completing other course work, it will ultimately be read and marked by another person who can only award a grade based on what you have written on the page, not what you intended to write! Furthermore, a poorly structured essay may not allow your ideas to shine through. This is a missed opportunity, as everything you wanted and intended to say has not found its way into your coursework and your excellent ideas have been wasted. So, in developing your written essay you should aim to tell a good story.

It is a good idea to ensure that you make clear connections between sentences and paragraphs so that the narrative flows. A useful technique here is to link your sentences by using joining words (or conjunctions) or phrases, such as:

- Furthermore. . .
- Additionally. . .
- In short. . .
- That is. . .
- So. . .
- Therefore. . .

For example, consider these sentences:

> These things must be considered when observing a client's vital signs – blood pressure, temperature, respiration and pulse.
>
> There are many things to consider when observing a client's vital signs. Blood pressure is very important, as is taking someone's pulse. Additionally, taking the client's temperature is essential. One must also ensure that respiration is noted.

Which one do you think has a better narrative flow?

Presentation of Written Work

It is easier to read a text that is well presented. Indeed, the ways in which you present the work will impact upon the overall mark you are awarded. Here, I offer you some advice concerning how to present your written work.

Headings and subheadings

Headings can be a useful way to develop the structure of your work, and can help you to present your work in a coherent and logical way. They can help both you and the reader to

navigate their way through your written work. You may think of them as signposts and t
work as a journey with a specific route to follow. Try to ensure that each heading relates
a specific theme, topic or issue. Subheadings can also be a useful aid to assist in subdividi
your work and providing more direction and structure. Be careful, though, in not using t
many headings and subheadings as this can seriously impact on the overall narrative flo
so if you are going to use them, ensure that they head a number of paragraphs. Howev
the use of headings is quite controversial and not all of your tutors will want you to u
them, so it may be as well to confirm that their use is acceptable!

You should always present headings and subheadings in a consistent manner. If you
using headings and subheadings, remember they should be typed in the same font st
throughout your work. It may be helpful to set yourself a guide as to the style of headin
and subheadings that you will use so that you use this consistently throughout all ye
academic work.

Paragraphs

Think carefully about paragraphing and how these are presented. Each paragraph sho
have only one theme. Paragraphs should contain more than one sentence but should
be too long; about two or three a page is preferable. Having a paragraph extending o
more than one page is too long. It you have too many concepts in one paragraph this
become confusing and extremely difficult for the marker to follow.

Within every paragraph each sentence will link ideas that relate to the theme. Make s
that every sentence is making one point that has not been said before. Each senten
should have its own discrete meaning that follows through ideas from the previous o
It can be easy to develop tautology (i.e. saying the same thing twice) and this should
avoided. Check that every sentence has a subject (e.g. 'I', 'You' and 'We'), a verb and
object (e.g. something the subject does something to) and never omit articles (i.e. 't
or 'a').

Repetition

The same words should not be repeated within the sentence. Preferably they should
be repeated in the subsequent or preceding sentences. This can be quite a challenge!
illustrate why this is problematic, consider the following:

> It is important to be careful when caring for a client, and we must adopt a caring approach t
> our care. So, it is important to take care in providing care.

You will find a thesaurus useful to find alternative words. Indeed, if you are word processing you will often find that your software has its own electronic thesaurus which can be very helpful.

Layout

When completing your work consider the finer details of presenting the overall layout of the text. You will be required to number the pages concurrently throughout the text. It is usual to present the text of academic work double spaced and type within the default margins of the page, that is, at least 2.4 cm margins on all sides on one side of an A4 page only. Leave a line between each paragraph.

Consider the use of bullet points carefully. Bullet points are useful if you are categorizing or listing points, for example in a report, but not in an essay that is developing critical arguments, so reduce your use of them to a minimum. They also have the habit of undermining narrative flow if they are over-used.

Standards and requirements in the presentation of written work can vary, so do ensure that you confirm the accepted style with your tutor or examine the 'house style' required by your university.

Developing Your Writing Style

Grammar, syntax, spelling and punctuation

It is important to follow the principles of standardized English grammar. Remember to check that punctuation marks such as full stops and commas are immediately at the end of the letter of the word and that there are no spaces in between unless you are designing the text in that way.

Be careful to use the apostrophe appropriately. For example, 'The student's notebook' means 'the notebook of the student' rather than 'The students' notebook', which means 'the notebook of more than one student'. Try also to remember that 'its' means 'belonging to it' whereas 'it's' is shorthand for 'it is'!

You will also need to consider your use of commas in a sentence and this can be quite complicated! Essentially, commas help you structure and break up a sentence. When you read your work out loud, commas are the point when you take a breath. This is why it is

helpful to say your work out aloud so that you check the spacing and punctuation ma
by the flow of your speech.

Ideally, abbreviations, colloquial expressions and slang words should be avoided in writ
professional language. They can also lead to confusion, as words used by lay people m
have different connotations from their clinical use. Slang words directed at disadvantag
or disabled people must *never* be used by professional people, in either written or ver
form. If you are using abbreviations such as initials for a title be careful in their use. O
use well accepted abbreviations such as Nursing and Midwifery Council (NMC) when y
have written the title out in full and placed the initials after this within parenthesis the f
time you use it.

Each time you write try to develop your use of words that are used in your field of pract
You will find a dictionary helpful to have at your side when writing. This will also help w
spelling words with which you are not familiar. Spelling will require special attentio
you are using the spell checker on the word processor as it does not pick up all errors.
example, the spell checker on your word processing software will say that the follow
sentence has no spelling mistakes:

> 'Nurses and midwives from an important part of health acre.'

If it does not make sense to you, it will not make sense to the reader.

So, there is no substitute for proof reading (and possibly re-reading) your completed w
(You may have noticed the problem with use of the word 'acre' instead of 'care' but did y
notice in the above sentence that the word 'form' should have be used instead of 'from'

Care needs to be taken to ensure that United Kingdom English is spelt rather than Ameri
or Australian English. Ensure that your spell checker is set to the correct form of Engl
Also remember to be consistent with spelling of words that may be spelt in more th
one way. For example: judgement, or judgment or organisation or organization. Fina
remember that even if you set the spell checker in your word processing software
Standard English it is unlikely to have correct words for technical healthcare language a
may interpret its own spelling.

Using quotations

Direct quotations must always be referenced with page numbers. Try not to use lo
quotations as it detracts from the analysis. If using a quotation there should be a writ

indication or a justification for its use and its relevance to the text either before or after using it. Use quotations carefully and try not to use them if you can develop the text yourself.

Quotations must be an accurate copy of the original. Replicate any underlining or italics in the original text but it is usual to indicate this in a note, such as 'original emphasis'. If you wish to emphasize part of a quotation by use of italics or underlining you need to indicate this in a note at the end of the quotation (e.g. 'emphasis added').

Longer quotations (e.g. of sentence length or more) should be indented from the default margin, and you must leave one space above and below the text. Such quotations can also be single spaced, to further illustrate that these are not your words. In writing a quotation, you may wish to edit out some words which are not relevant to your purposes. Here, you should use three full stops as dots to indicate that you have removed some words, that is '. . .' This is called an ellipsis.

You may also wish to add further points of clarification to your text. Footnotes or endnotes may be used where appropriate, but are not usually used in undergraduate assignments. You will need to ask your tutor about use of appendices. These are additions that clarify the written text and are usually only used in long assignments such as reports or dissertations.

When English Isn't Your First Language

You are strongly advised to seek help from your learning support services at your university if you feel that you lack fluency or confidence in your verbal or written English. Do make use of these services as you will not do justice to your ideas, or obtain the grades you deserve if you are not able to communicate effectively. It will also be most helpful if you a have a friend who understands fluent English and who is willing to read through the text of some of your written work before submission so that it is corrected. This may be a person who is not familiar with the profession as they can look at the presentation with fresh eyes and provide you with guidance on the grammar and the sense of your English.

There are also very helpful books on the market for students who have English as a second language that give details of how to present your written text in a grammatical way. Common errors that occur for students who do not have English as their first language are the use of the personal pronouns (such as 'I', 'You' and 'They') and deciding when it is appropriate to use them, and the use of tenses.

Another area where there is often confusion is when to use the definite article 'the' and the indefinite article 'a' in front of nouns. For example, the following sentence is a typical example of someone who is not fluent in their use of written English: 'If patient has chest infection you observe rapid breathing.' Correctly, the sentence might be written like this 'If *a* patient has *a* chest infection *then* you *may* observe rapid breathing.'

Remember, 'the' client refers to a specific client whereas 'a' client refers to any client. Some languages do not have this convention (or make as much use of articles as English), and can seem rather strange if you are not used to it.

A Final Thought

Each person has their own style and gifts of writing and thinking. Thinking about and planning each piece of work before you write and taking the time to consider the feedback given when it is returned to you will assist your future planning and help you to develop your ability to write in an academic way.

Tips

- Think through the plan of your work before you begin to write
- Always read your work through after writing it
- Always have a good dictionary with you when you write to ensure that you develop your use of new words
- Use a thesaurus so that you limit the number of repetitions of words that you are using and develop your vocabulary.

Reference

Benner, P. (1984) *From Novice to Expert: Excellence and Power in Clinical Nursing Practice.* Menlo Park, California, Addison-Wesley.

Chapter 13

How to Reference and Avoid Plagiarism

by David Stroud

This chapter addresses:

- **Why accurate and systematic referencing is an important academic issue**

- **The basics of accurate referencing**

- **What paraphrasing is and how to use direct quotations**

- **What primary and secondary referencing are**

- **How to compile a reference list**

- **What plagiarism is, and how to avoid it.**

Introduction

In this chapter you will be offered guidance on how to reference accurately and systematically. It will make you aware of what plagiarism actually means and the importance acknowledging other people's work and ideas. Each university has a slightly different s of requirements when it comes to referencing, and the first step is to ensure that you ha these guidelines available, and that you understand them fully. You will need to refer ba to these guidelines regularly when you compose your theoretical assessments, so ke them safe and to hand! In this chapter, I will offer you broad advice to ensure that y understand the basic principles to avoid plagiarism.

Why Reference?

Academic work requires you to make it possible for the reader to track down any quotatio or ideas you have used. This is achieved through the accurate use of an accepted referencin system. In this way, readers can verify the authenticity of your work and follow up anythin of particular interest to them. Referencing is also a way of giving authors the credit th they deserve. Another reason to reference is to say to the marker, 'Hey, look at the amou of work I put into this!'

Remember that attention to detail in referencing is as important as the content of yo work. Referencing should not be seen as an add-on to your essay but integral to the over academic presentation of your work. Valuable marks can be lost through poor referencin and it could easily make the difference between a pass and a referral/fail.

Markers are experts in their particular subject area. They are often fully aware of t important literature in their field. Therefore, when marking an assignment, non-reference or inaccurately referenced work can often be easily recognized. If there is a suspicion th literature has been used or copied extensively in an essay, and without appropriate cre to the author, then this can lead to an investigation and possible disciplinary action.

What to Reference

You are required to reference all sources of words or ideas that you use in your assignmen These sources may be, for instance, books, journals, Internet, newspapers, person communications, TV programmes, websites or conference proceedings. You must al acknowledge unpublished material in exactly the same way as published material.

Your references should be as up to date as possible. An exception to this general rule is if it is considered a 'seminal' piece of work. Seminal comes from the Latin word *semin*, to germinate or sow. Bulls used for that purpose in Spain are called *seminales*! There is no limit on the age of such references – you could find yourself referencing Hippocrates (400 BC) on his theory of personality or 'temperaments'. Some examples of seminal work that you might come across in health care are Maslow (1970) hierarchy of needs, Hans Seyle (1946) theory of stress, McCaffrey (1968) pain theory and Kubler-Ross (1970) stages of grief.

How to Reference

The most common referencing methods are the Harvard system (or author-date system), the Vancouver system (or number system) and the Footnotes method. The Harvard system is more commonly used in nursing and midwifery literature, and will be most likely the referencing style you will be asked to adopt. The Vancouver system is usually favoured in the scientific or medical literature. The Footnotes method is a less used method which involves putting a number in the text indicating the reference at the foot of the page. Have you noticed which system is used in this book?

There can be slight variations in the use of the Harvard system between universities, or even between one faculty and another, so before starting work on your assignments, make sure you obtain the official guidelines from your faculty or university department. Follow them meticulously and ensure that your referencing is both accurate and consistent throughout the text and your reference list.

The following examples highlight the basics of referencing using the Harvard system. Please note this is not an exhaustive list.

An authored book

Imagine you were writing an essay on the nervous system. You might write something like this:

> There are in fact, not one but two nervous systems – one that we can control voluntarily and one that functions automatically (Campbell 2003).

Here, you are backing up your claim that the body has a voluntary and autonomic nervous system by making reference to John Campbell's excellent book on physiology. As you have

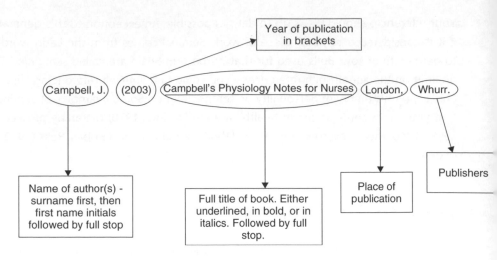

Figure 13.1   An authored book.

cited Campbell in the text of your essay you will now need to record this in a reference ▶ which will be located at the end of your essay using the format described in Figure 13.1

As you can see, there is a very structured way to record your references. If the book h been authored by more than one person, then you will cite each author in the order th they appear on the book cover.

There can be some variations to the above format. For example, the book title must highlighted by using either a bold font, underlining or italicizing. Sometimes the name the publishers is placed before the place of publication, sometimes vice versa. This i matter of the 'house style' that your university will adopt and they will inform you abc their required format.

An edited book

The above book was written by an author. However, some books, such as the one you reading, are edited books. An edited book is a collection of work (divided into chapte written by different authors. Here, if you are citing an author you are referring in the fi instance to their chapter, which is located within a book. Your reference list will need record this. So, imagine you were writing an essay on the working with carers of serv users with mental health problems. You might write something like this:

> There is a need for mental health professionals to consider not only the needs of the service users, but also the needs of carers as well (Jones 2005).

Jones (2005) is the author of a chapter in an edited book, and Figure 13.2 illustrates how this should be recorded in your reference list.

A journal article

It is likely that you will want to cite articles written in journals. Imagine you were writing about the sort of knowledge that nurses might use in their clinical practice. You might write something like this:

> There are, it seems, a number of types of knowledge which are fundamental to nursing/midwifery practice – science, art, an understanding of morality and our own personal knowledge (Carper 1978).

Carper (1978) is a seminal work which highlights the complexity of nursing knowledge, and Figure 13.3 illustrates how this should be recorded.

Direct Quotations

If you are making reference to another person's work, you will most commonly 'paraphrase' which simply means rewriting an idea, comment or research finding in your own words. It ensures that you really understand what you have read and how it relates to your topic. You must ensure that you cite the author of any work you have paraphrased, to ensure that you are giving the author the appropriate credit.

However, you can also use 'direct quotations' and this is when you cite the words that an author uses in their own work. Often you will choose to quote directly when an author uses a significant or memorable phrase that you believe captures the point you wish to make. Sometimes, an author expresses an idea so poignantly and precisely that you feel paraphrasing would undermine some of its potency. Take, for example, this quote:

> How could we understand how someone has become sunk into despair, or a prisoner of their fears, or persecuted by voices, unless we are prepared to be a compassionate presence in their search for meaning in the psychological, social, spiritual and bodily dimensions of their experience? (Watkins, 2001, p. 45).

As you can see, in addition to citing the author and year of publication in your text, you also need to cite the page number where this quote can be located – in this example, in Watkins (2001) on page 45. When you use direct quotes, you must be careful to duplicate the exact words the author has used and always enclose direct quotes in inverted commas unless the quote is taken out of the text and displayed indented, usually in a smaller typeface.

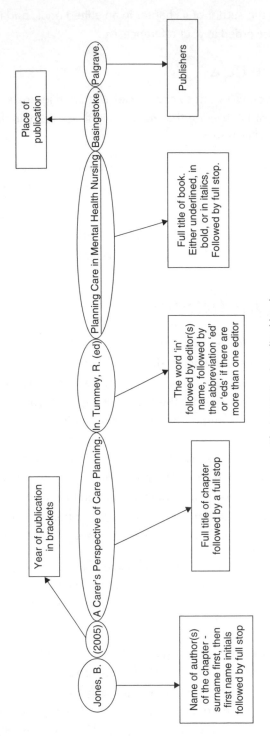

Figure 13.2   An edited book.

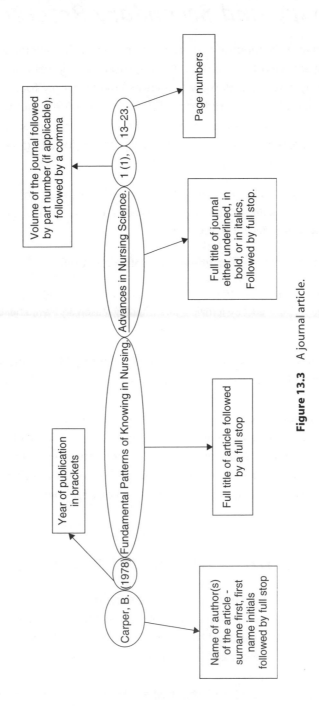

Figure 13.3   A journal article.

Primary and Secondary Referencing

As a student, it is important for you to understand the difference between primary a
secondary sources of information. If you cite from the original work of a writer, this is know
as a primary reference. Primary references are commonly found, but not exclusively,
research journals or authored books. If, however, you cite an author whose work is *referr*
to in another source, such as textbooks, then this is a secondary reference. And you ha
probably guessed this by now, there is a protocol for citing secondary references! F
example, you might write:

> According to Bowlby (1969 cited by Mason and Whitehead 2003) new born children are
> genetically programmed to become attached or 'bonded' to a female figure. This theory has
> generated much debate in recent years.

You could also express this differently if you would prefer:

> According to Bowlby (1969), new born children are genetically programmed to become
> attached or 'bonded' to a female figure (cited by Mason and Whitehead 2003). This theory has
> generated much debate in recent years.

In your reference list, you would record the work by Mason and Whitehead (2003) on
That is, secondary referenced work is not recorded in your reference list.

It is good academic discipline to try hard to seek out the primary sources. Don't overu
secondary references, particularly when they are obtained easily from your library or onli
electronic database. You would only use secondary references if the work is difficult
obtain, such as being long out of print. The problem with secondary references is that th
are often an interpretation of an author's work by another writer and something may
lost in translation.

Completing Your Reference List

Your reference list, which will be a separate section of your essay and will follow on from th
text of your theoretical assignment, is the way in which you collate the work of the autho
you have cited. It is essential to compile your reference list accurately and systematica
and in alphabetical order according to authors' names.

Students often get confused about what date to use when referencing a book that h
been revised or reprinted. You should use the *copyright* date of the most recent editi

(indicated by the copyright symbol ©), not any reprint dates, and these details should be taken from the book's title page and its reverse title page. Some books display this information more clearly than others! If for any reason a publication date is not stated for a work, then n.d. (no date) should be written in your reference list. Write n.p. (no place) if the place of publication is not available.

Don't forget, when you are writing your essays, to keep a detailed record of all the references that you use to facilitate the writing up of your reference list.

Producing a Bibliography

While all your written assignments must have a reference section, a bibliography is normally optional and, unless specifically asked for, will not usually be marked. A bibliography is a record of all the background or preparatory reading for a theoretical assessment, which is not referred to in your assignment. It is compiled in exactly the same way as your reference list.

What is Plagiarism?

Putting forward another person's thoughts and using their words is perfectly acceptable as long as they are properly acknowledged. Plagiarism, however, is defined as passing off another's work as your own, either intentionally or unintentionally, and the failure to acknowledge the source of any material used in your academic assignments. However, this can be any other person's work not only published authors; it may be fellow students' essays, or handouts and lecture notes. Unless sufficient care is taken, it can be easy to take an idea from a published work and include it without appropriate acknowledgement.

Even though plagiarism can be committed quite innocently, it can still incur serious penalties. Universities give clear guidance on how you can avoid plagiarizing work and have stringent policies to enforce their regulations.

The word comes from the Latin for kidnapper, *plagiarius*, and today it denotes any kind of intellectual theft. But there is no easy way of saying it. Whether there is a deliberate intention to pass off another's work as one's own or not, plagiarism is cheating which may have serious implications for your future career.

It is important, therefore, that you take steps to avoid being accused of plagiarism. If y are accused of plagiarism, you will need to prove the authenticity of your work and th you are the author. Follow any guidance issued by your university, but in addition I wou advise that you keep copies of notes and essay plans to demonstrate how you planne developed and constructed your assignment. It would also be useful to keep copies journal articles and other cited literature and be prepared to discuss how this work help you to develop your ideas.

Group Work

You are sometimes encouraged, or even directed, to work in small groups. That is, you m be required to undertake work of a collaborative nature. It is not unusual for univers students to work together on their assignments. There are definite advantages to th such as the promotion of teamwork and sharing ideas and information. However, wh the aim is for each individual student to submit an individual piece of work resulting fro their group activities, it is essential that you make sure that no part of your work is exac the same as that of any of your fellow students.

Final Thoughts

Remember that if you are still unsure about anything, seek clarification on referen ing and plagiarism issues from your personal tutor or the Plagiarism Advisory Servi (www.jiscpas.ac.uk) which is there to give you further advice and guidance.

Tips

Keep detailed records of all references you use.

- To avoid too closely reflecting phrases or ideas from the original, don't base your ess on only one or two sources
- Ensure that you follow any guidance issued by your university in relation to referenci and plagiarism
- Try to limit your secondary references
- Keep all your essay plans and copies of drafts too if you are required to demonstra authenticity.

References

Campbell, J. (2003) *Campbell's Physiology Notes for Nurses.* London, Whurr.

Carper, B. (1978) Fundamental patterns of knowing in nursing. *Advances in Nursing Science* **1**(1), 13–23.

Jones B. (2005) A carer's perspective of care planning. In Tummey R. (ed). Planning Care in Mental Health Nursing. Basingstoke, Palgrave.

Kubler-Ross, E. (1970) *On Death and Dying.* London, Tavistock Publications.

Maslow, A. (1970) *Motivation and Personality.* London, Harper Collins.

Mason, T. and Whitehead, E. (2003) *Thinking Nursing.* Maidenhead, Open University Press.

McCaffrey, M. (1968) *Cognition, Bodily Pain and Man/Environmental Interactions.* Los Angeles, University of California Student Store.

Seyle, H. (1946) The general adaptation syndrome and the diseases of adaptation. *J Clin Endocrinol. Metab.,* 6, 117–230.

Watkins, P. (2001) *Mental Health Nursing: the Art of Compassionate Care.* Edinburgh, Butterworth Heinemann.

References

Chapter 14

Making the Most of Assessment Feedback

by Lai Chan Koh

This chapter considers:

- **What assessment feedback is**
- **How to plan getting feedback**
- **What to ask about feedback**
- **How to make the most of feedback in practice areas.**

Introduction

Following each of your assessments throughout your programme, you will receive feedba
which is aimed at helping you to enhance your learning and improve your performar
in future assessments. Good feedback tells you what is expected, how well you are do
and what you might need to change to develop yourself in your academic work or clini
practice. It acts as a stimulus and should give you the confidence to develop your work. A
consequence, you will grow as a student and practitioner, and knowledge of your strengt
as well as limitations, helps you to develop a positive self-concept while improving yo
self-esteem. Belief in yourself that you have the ability to succeed motivates you to s
focused on the assessment task.

Feedback should be seen as an integral part of your learning and professional developme
This chapter explains how to make the most of assessment feedback.

What is Assessment Feedback?

On your programme you will be assessed in your theory and in your practice, and for ea
of the assessments you should receive feedback on how well you have done. Assessme
feedback is commentary made about the standard of your assessed work in light
the required learning outcomes. It is given in different forms – verbal, written, electror
individual, group and so forth, and lets you know what you are good at (your strength
and what your developmental needs are (your weaknesses). To help you to know wh
you are and where you need to be, the feedback includes suggestions of what further w
is to be done so as to attain greater achievement.

Feedback relates not just to the healthcare subjects that you study, but also to
skills such as communication (oral and written), information technology, application
numbers, problem solving, teamwork and professional development, which are of
important considerations for many employers.

There are two types of feedback, one that follows a 'formative' assessment and the otl
a 'summative' assessment. A formative assessment is an ongoing process where y
learning progress is assessed. A summative assessment is a final assessment and usu
occurs towards the end of the module/unit of study and will be marked and graded.
mark will be the basis on which a decision is made on whether or not you can progress
the programme.

Normally, for a formative assessment, no mark or grade is given. However, you can expect feedback from such an assessment, which can be given informally by your peers and/or your tutor. For example, you might by offered advice or comments following your oral presentation of a project.

This feedback is usually given verbally. Sometimes you are given written feedback from your tutor that serves as an authoritative external reference point against which you can evaluate your progress. Another way of helping you to learn via feedback is by engaging in online learning activities such as multiple choice questions and discussion via electronic learning resources, such as 'Blackboard', which can be accessed any time, any place and as many times as you wish.

The focus of formative feedback is on your learning. It is for you and your peers to assess each other's work in a supportive way. Apart from raising awareness of your communication skills, the experience is beneficial because your peers challenge your knowledge and beliefs and expose you to alternative perspectives and strategies. This enables you to construct new knowledge and meaning. This process helps you to understand the defined criteria, encourages you to reflect on your learning and enables you to review and self-adjust your work in order to meet the standards of your assessment. It is essential to participate in classroom activities and get feedback.

As you develop and hone your skills and knowledge using feedback, you will become less dependent on others to assess and to tell you where you are going wrong (and where you are going right as well). By this stage, you become actively involved in monitoring and regulating your own performance both in terms of goals and in terms of the strategies being used to reach those goals. This is the process that develops you as a lifelong learner and one that helps you develop confidence in yourself as a practitioner.

Understanding What is Expected

At the beginning of your programme, it is not always easy to grasp the academic standard required of you. An approach that has proved particularly powerful in clarifying what is expected is the use of 'exemplars' of good performance. Exemplars are effective because they define an objective and valid standard against which you can compare your work. You may wish to look at some of these exemplars to help you to achieve greater understanding of the assessment requirements.

How to Plan Getting Feedback

When formative feedback is given, it is important that you take time to reflect on comments that have been made. The process involves you actively in the generation plan for your own personal and professional development.

When you receive feedback following your summative assessment, again take time reflect on comments made. It might be that you have not done so well as you would h wanted, or indeed might have to resubmit your work as it was not up to the stand required. You should ensure that you see your tutor, or other appropriate person, to disc the feedback as soon as possible so that you give yourself enough time to rewrite y work without rushing to meet deadlines. It is important to ensure that you are receptive such feedback – it can be difficult sometimes, even painful, to hear what we might se negative comments about us and we might be tempted to become defensive and re such comments. However, try to put this in context – the only purpose of well intentior constructive feedback is to help you to succeed in your chosen programme.

To help you to make the best use of the time with your tutor, some preparation is necess before the meeting. You can start by reading your assessed work again and revisiting assessment guidelines stated in your module document. I would then suggest reading marker's feedback comments carefully in order to make sense of what is said about areas you need to improve upon. When listing the key questions to ask your tutor, these in order, with the most important first, in case you run out of time and do not through the list.

Finally, you will need to prepare an outline of your proposed action plan. If you do straight on to the computer, you can reorganize the plan on screen, and progressiv build on this. Take this plan with you to the meeting so that your tutor knows what you trying to do and gives further direction.

It may be necessary for you to meet your tutor more than once if you feel that you n further guidance. Alternatively, you may wish to discuss online the development of y work. Sometimes, a group tutorial is arranged to give you and other students additic support. Equally, I would suggest trying to develop your own support networks with y peers with whom you can discuss ideas, difficulties and find out how they have approac similar problems.

If it has been identified that you need support with development of some of your key skills such as communication or application of number and information technology, you may be referred to a Learning Support Unit where you can get specific help with these skills. Seeking and obtaining support following feedback can make a real difference to the standard of your work.

What to Ask About Feedback

Knowing what questions to ask about your feedback is the starting process of improving and developing your academic skills and improving on your assessed work. However, knowing what to ask means that you have made sense of the comments and formulated questions of both your work and the feedback. This is important as the feedback must be interpreted and internalized before you can take further action to adjust your work. If you do not understand the feedback comments, ask for clarification. You can also seek guidance on further reading that is recommended to develop your thinking and to improve your work.

So, the aim of clarification is to seek shared understanding between you and your tutor of the assessment criteria and the required standard. If you don't share your tutor's understanding of the assessment requirements, then the feedback information you receive is unlikely to 'connect' with you. In this case, it will be difficult for you to evaluate gaps between your actual and the required performance.

Although the mark reflects the overall standard of your work, the feedback normally has comments relevant to a specific standard using a set of marking criteria or descriptors. Examples of these criteria are structure and presentation of your work; content; analysis, synthesis and evaluation; your use of literature and quality of referencing; and clarity of expression.

The comments on structure identify how your ideas are presented, whether it shows any coherence. Further, it is necessary in academic essays to have a clear introduction and a firm conclusion. A clear structure helps your assessors to find their way through ideas and arguments that are detailed and logically developed. If they can't see what you're doing, or why your arguments are relevant, they cannot give you many marks.

Feedback on content relates to the extent to which the required aims of the assessment have been addressed. This is often a reflection of the quality of your literature searches and the information you use to underpin arguments. You should aim to read widely as it will help you to develop depth and breadth of your knowledge. As for analysis, synthesis and evaluation, feedback comments highlight your ability to demonstrate higher level thinking and to think 'outside the box'. Your assessor will also be looking for a clear line of reasoning and how every example and piece of information contributes to that line of reasoning.

Comments on the use of literature point to the evidence that is used to explain your thinking and how you arrive at your opinion. In other words, the evidence of reading that is used to support your arguments or discussion. The evidence has to be explained rather than described so as to convince the assessor of the relevance of the ideas selected from your reading. The explanation also demonstrates that you are not accepting ideas uncritically and without question.

In order to help the assessor to understand your work, you need to use the correct words and phrases that will convey them accurately. Therefore correct paragraphing, grammar, punctuation, spelling and your overall writing style are important aspects of academic writing with entitlement to higher grades. The quality of your academic writing is also influenced by the way your work is referenced. It shows your understanding of the reading and its effective use to back up your arguments or claims.

Moreover, you must follow the referencing system required by your university. Thus, before you submit your work, it is good practice to proof read it to amend any grammatical and spelling errors and to check that the referencing is correct and consistent. This can improve your presentation and can make a difference to your overall mark.

If your assessment is an examination, your assessed work is often not returned to you. However, you can ask to look at it and you should ensure that you obtain feedback, particularly if you have to retake the examination. Again, it will be useful to read the assessment guidelines and marking criteria in advance prior to discussing the feedback with your tutor. If the assessment consists of multiple choice questions or short questions, review the questions and answers and ask why incorrect answers are wrong. If the feedback highlights your management of time for the examination needs special attention, it is worth while spending time to practise writing under examination conditions.

Your programme assessment may include a portfolio. This kind of assessment requires you to show evidence of achievement as a record of ongoing development over time. Examples of such evidence include reflective accounts, concept maps, reports, summaries, leaflets is aimed at encouraging you to identify your own standard by evaluating your own work and offering you the opportunity to be creative and go beyond the essential requirement of your study. Again, it is important to ask for feedback on the correct interpretation of the assessment requirements, whether you have submitted the essential evidence and whether the work is acceptable in terms of its overall presentation.

How to Make the Most of Assessment in the Practice Area

Nursing and midwifery programmes require you to be assessed in practice as well as in theory. In the practical assessment, you have to demonstrate that you have achieved the specified learning outcomes related to the development of your clinical practice.

In each practice area, you will be supervised by a mentor whose role is to support your clinical learning and assess your performance as a practitioner. This support should include identifying your learning needs at the start of your practice experience, planning learning opportunities, instilling self-confidence in your practice and, finally, assessing you. As an adult learner, you should also be helped to connect your learning to real life experiences, in other words, to integrate your theoretical knowledge with clinical practice.

The practical assessment, like the theoretical assessment, has formative and summative components. Formative feedback is ongoing and will be given throughout the period of your experience in that placement. Sometimes, if you think that you are not getting sufficient feedback, you should ensure that you ask for it. Do not assume that you are making the necessary progress because your mentor has not given you feedback! At the mid-point of your experience, your mentor will discuss your learning in more detail and you will be given oral and written feedback of your progress. Just like the feedback of your theoretical assessment, comments will be made about your strengths and your weaknesses, but will be focused mainly on your practice.

The feedback from your mentor is centred on your knowledge, skills and attitude (performance, technical skills and behaviours) based on direct observation of your clinical practice. Try to make sense of the feedback, build on your strong points and take time to understand the areas that need further development. Your mentor will guide you on what experiences and learning opportunities you should focus on to improve your performance. You may also be advised to read on certain subjects relevant to your practice and your mentor will be looking for your ability to integrate theory with practice.

At the end of your placement, your mentor will complete a summative assessment of y
achievement. The written feedback will highlight your strengths and areas that still requ
further development. This information should be noted and used to prepare you for y
next placement. This is of particular importance if you are required to do the assessm
again.

Conclusion

Feedback is given following formative and summative assessments. To make the m
of your assessment feedback, you need to plan how to get feedback and to know w
to ask. If this approach is adopted following each theoretical and practical assessm
assessment feedback can enhance your learning and enable you to attain better grade

Tips

- Be clear what is required of you before you commence your assessment
- Try to see feedback in positive terms – try not to become defensive
- Read your feedback comments carefully
- If you are unsure about any of the comments relating to formative or summa
  assessments, then seek clarification.

Section 3

Developing Clinical Skills

In this section, the focus is on helping you to develop clinical skills necessary for modern healthcare practice.

Many students consider this part of their programme to be the most enjoyable and the most rewarding. However, it is important to consider how you might prepare, develop and enhance your clinical skills both while you are undertaking the practice part of your programme, and also while at your university. Thus it is important to consider how you take full advantage of skills laboratories in your university and how you might then seek out learning opportunities in clinical practice.

Chapter 15

Maximizing Your Learning in Practice Placements

by Karen Elcock and Stella Brophy

This chapter considers:

- **Roles and responsibilities of key people involved in your learning in practice placements**
- **What preparation to undertake before commencing your placement**
- **Strategies for getting the most from your placement**
- **Maximizing your learning opportunities**
- **How to learn on placement**
- **Self-assessment**
- **Evaluating practice learning.**

Introduction

Going out on placement is probably the most enjoyable but also the most daunting p
of your programme. It also plays an important part in your learning. A placement is wh
you will gain direct experience of care, under supervision, in a range of different prac
environments, such as acute hospitals, the community and independent, voluntary a
social care sectors. During this time you will be able to apply theory to practice and le
new theories based on your experiences in the placement.

You will have many opportunities to practise and develop a range of skills and to acqu
the professional attributes expected of a registered nurse or midwife. This can all be qu
challenging as you will also be studying for academic assessments at the same time a
trying to have a personal life!

However, most students say that their time in placements is the best part of the program
You must remember that you are not going out on placement to work but to learn. Learn
on your placement is different from learning in the university, so this chapter offers so
ideas on how you can get the best from your time on placement.

Clarifying Roles, Expectations and Responsibilities in Clinical Practice

On your practice placements, clinical staff will have expectations of you in terms of y
professional presentation and behaviour. Your university will also have a set of regulati
which you will be expected to adhere to. This means that you will be required to arr
punctually at the practice placement, dressed neatly and appropriately and have attenc
to your personal hygiene.

While on placement you will come into contact with a large number and diverse rar
of people including healthcare professionals, patients/clients, mothers, babies and
public in general. This can be quite overwhelming! However, there are key people availa
to support you while on placement, in particular your mentor and lecturers from
university. But do remember that your personal tutor and other academic staff at
university are still available for help and support.

A mentor is a registered nurse, midwife or public health professional who has undertak
a recognized programme to prepare them for their role. Every student is allocate

mentor but you may also be allocated an associate mentor (often called a co-mentor), who provides support when your mentor is not available. However, it is the duty of all qualified nurses and midwives to 'facilitate students of nursing, midwifery. . . and others to develop their competence' (NMC 2004a, clause 6.4).

Your mentor is there to facilitate learning opportunities for you, to act as a resource and will assess you on your competencies in your practice assessment document. The Nursing and Midwifery Council (NMC) advises that mentors should spend at least 40% of their time with the student (about two days per week) but that does not necessarily mean that they will be glued to your side as they have other responsibilities. Indeed, it is important to remember that your mentor will always prioritize patient care above your needs.

Other members of the team are also there to support you while on placement and they will all discuss your progress with your mentor so that a fair assessment can be made at the end of your placement. Some universities have a lecturer who acts as the link between the university and practice. They provide support to mentors and students, monitor the quality of the environment for learning by undertaking educational audits and act as a resource to practice staff. Other people who also support learners and mentors on placement are practice educators, lecturer practitioners, clinical placement facilitators and practice education facilitators. Each National Health Service (NHS) trust and university will have a slightly different way of working, so it is always best to seek information about available support from your university or mentor.

One of the main reasons for difficulties arising from clinical problems is confusion about roles, responsibilities and expectations. Table 15.1 gives an overview of what you can expect and what will be expected of you. It is useful to check these out with your mentor each time you start a new placement.

Supernumerary Status

Your status as a 'supernumerary' student is still poorly understood, so let's get it straight!

All pre-registration students have supernumerary status while on placement for their whole programme. The Royal College of Nursing (RCN 2002, p.20) describes supernumerary status as follows:

> students are additional to the workforce requirements and staffing establishment figures. However, they must make a contribution to the work of the practice area to enable them to learn how to care for patients.

Table 15.1   Expectations related to your learning on placement

What you can expect	What will be expected of you
A supportive learning environment	You have prepared for the placement and ha contacted them in advance
An orientation to your placement and health and safety issues discussed	You follow the NMC Code of Professional Conduct (NMC 2004a) and Guidelines for Students of Nursing and Midwifery (NMC 2002)
Respect for your supernumerary status	You take an active approach to your studies, negotiating with your mentor to access appropriate learning opportunities and to complete practice assessments
Time to discuss your learning needs, agree a plan for learning and agree dates for review	You work collaboratively with members of th multidisciplinary team to the benefit of patients and clients across the range of sh patterns in the practice area
Access to appropriate experiences and resources to facilitate your learning as a health professional	You are aware of and follow policies and procedures within the Trust/practice environment
Support from a mentor/assessor who will provide guidance on an ongoing basis through a placement experience	You acknowledge your own limitations and s clarification and supervision as appropria
Feedback from practice staff on your progress and ongoing learning needs	You are punctual, appropriately dressed and professionally at all times
Experience which will help you to achieve the expected learning outcomes	You evaluate your practice experience with constructive comments
An opportunity to evaluate your practice experience with knowledge that these comments will be acted upon	

The last sentence is important. You need to take part in the care of clients/patie if you are to learn; it is also important if you want to be accepted by the clin staff. Unlike the old apprenticeship system where students were relied upon as p of the workforce, supernumerary status gives you the opportunity to access learn opportunities because the staff are not reliant on you as 'an extra pair of hands'. In rea there will be occasions, which cannot be planned for, when the area is very busy a where clinical staff may need your help and this will be appreciated. This can also prov you with valuable learning opportunities. However, if you feel your supernumerary sta is being abused talk to your mentor, the manager in the placement or someone from university.

Preparation Before Commencing Placement

To get the most from your time on placement you will need to undertake some preparation before you start. This should start as soon as your university informs you where you are going for your placement. Remember a prepared student impresses clinical staff as it shows interest and motivation.

Where are you going?

Find out as much as you can about where you are going. Good sources of information are websites. Hospitals, primary care trusts and many independent and voluntary organizations have their own websites and many universities now have information about the placements on their own website. They will give you basic information about the organization, such as location and travel directions, but you will also find information about what you can expect to learn there.

Making contact with the placement

It is important to make contact with the placement prior to starting. Preferably try to arrange to visit them before you start. Questions you may wish to ask are:

- What type of placement is it and what experiences will they be able to offer you?
- What are the shift patterns?
- What is the expected dress code? Do you need to wear a uniform?
- Is there any recommended reading or activities you should undertake before you start?
- Can you visit in advance to meet your mentor, discuss your learning needs and off duty requirements? It is important to note that if you do visit your placement in advance you may have to wait to see your mentor or the manager if it is busy, so allow extra time.

Planning your learning

Once you have information about your placement you can start to plan your learning. Updating yourself by researching relevant clinical issues or the possible specialist focus of the practice area, and reviewing relevant reports from the Department of Health is a good start, as well as looking at what learning outcomes you will need to achieve on t placement.

If you have already been on placements before reflect on what went well and what not go so well. What were your strengths and weaknesses? Were areas identified that y needed to improve on? If so make a note of them. Identify which learning outcomes y feel confident about and those that you are unclear or worried about. All these areas can discussed with your mentor at your first meeting. Remember if you don't tell your mer about your weaknesses or worries he/she cannot help you to improve in those areas.

Maximizing Learning Opportunities

The initial interview

At this interview you will identify your learning needs with your mentor and agree a plar meet them. It is helpful to be clear about what the mentor will expect you to demonstr in order to meet the learning outcomes in your practice assessment. A useful way to this is to break down each learning outcome into three areas of learning (see Table 1 for an example) you will then know what you need to do to demonstrate achievemen the learning outcomes.

Table 15.2   Learning to be demonstrated in medicine administration

Knowledge	Skills	Attitude
NMC Guidelines for the Administration of Medicines (NMC 2004b)	Calculate correct dosage	Demonstrates motivation and interest by preparing for medicine administration in advance
Knowledge of medicines (agree which ones)	Safe dispensing of medicine	Demonstrates professional behaviour by adherence to medicine policy
For example action, side-effects, contraindications and interactions	Safe administration of medicines	Respects patient choice and autonomy
What action to take if patient cannot/will not take the medicine	Ensures medicines administered are recorded	Asks questions where unsure of knowledge
What observations to take before or after the medicine	Observation skills	Treats patients and staff with respect
	Communication skills	

Table 15.3   Activities to be undertaken to achieve competence in medicine administration

Knowledge	Skills	Attitude
Read NMC Guidelines for the Administration of Medicines (NMC 2004b)	Observe medicine round (×2)	Requests opportunity to practise medicine rounds at start of shift
Look up the medicines you have agreed to focus on in the *British National Formulary*	Undertake medicine round (under supervision) (×3)	Requests feedback on performance
Talk to patients about their views of the medicines they are on		
Arrange to meet with the pharmacist who visits your placement area		

This will form part of your learning contract between you and your mentor with an agreed action plan (see Table 15.3 for an example of activities you might undertake to achieve competence in medicine administration).

By having an agreed action plan, you can start each day on placement with a clear idea of what you want to achieve that day. Think of it as a type of shopping list of activities you want or need to do. At the start of each shift make sure you let people know what you want to do or see so that they can organize that within the schedule of activities for the day and can ensure you are given opportunities to achieve your learning outcomes.

Mid-point interview

Midway through your placement, it is important that you arrange to meet with your mentor to discuss your progress. Use your agreed action plan to review what has been achieved and what else you need to do. If there are areas you need to improve upon these must be highlighted by your mentor at the meeting and an action plan to help you make that improvement agreed between you. Remember it is up to you to remind your mentor that this meeting needs to take place.

Final interview

At the end of your placement you will review your learning with your mentor and complete your practice assessment documentation. It is important at this point to identify areas of both strength and weakness so that you know what you need to focus on in your next placement.

How to Learn on Placement

Placements offer a rich resource for learning. The following are just some of the ways t
you can achieve your learning outcomes.

Role modelling

Observing practitioners undertake care activities is the most common way of learni
However, just watching someone only allows you to learn *how* to do something but y
also need to know *why*. So ask questions. Why did they do that? What prompted t
course of action? What will happen next?

Learning skills

To learn a skill you will need to first observe a more experienced person undertake it. Y
will then need to practise it under supervision, and to develop proficiency further in t
skill you need to continue to practise it in different situations. If your university has a clin
skills centre you may wish to go back there to practise skills in a safe environment bef
practising on a patient/client.

Using handovers

At the start of each shift a handover is given from the staff just finishing their shift to
staff just starting. This is a valuable time for learning. Make a note of all the words you h
and don't understand and look them up or discuss with a member of staff.

Ask to attend multiprofessional team meetings and listen to what is being said. Mak
note of points you don't understand. Observe how members of the team communic
with the patient and the patient's response. What can you learn from this?

Providing patient care

You must always ask permission from a patient before undertaking any care with then
the patient does not want a student to provide care for them they have the right to refu
However, most patients are very willing to help you to learn. Patients today are far m
informed than in the past and so can give you useful information about their conditi
You can learn a lot by asking them how they first came to access the healthcare syst
and the treatment they have received. Ask them about their experiences, medications th
are on and how they have been affected. Learning about different conditions from a bo

might be complex, but learning about them from the patient's perspective means you are far more likely to remember. Likewise, learning about medications in relation to a specific patient will make far more sense than trying to memorize a list of them.

So, you might like to try this. Select one person you have been caring for. Read through their notes and care plans carefully in order to gain insight into their history. Next, ask the patient questions about their health difficulties and the care they have received. Find out what medications they are taking and any treatment they are receiving. Look up the anatomy, physiology and the pathophysiology or other issues that might be relevant to their health problem. Now, ensure that you reflect on what you have found and where you don't understand any areas talk to your mentor or tutor.

Learning from other members of the multidisciplinary team (MDT)

You will meet a whole range of other health and social care professionals during your programme. Understanding the role they play is important. You can do this by asking to shadow them at work, asking them questions about their role and getting involved in multidisciplinary team (MDT) meetings when out on placement. For example, you might like to observe the physiotherapist assisting a stroke patient with posture and balance, and then follow up that patient by accompanying him/her to the gym for further input or accompanying a patient/client to X-ray/body scanner.

Learning from peers

Each student will have a different set of experiences through their programme so your peers also have something to offer you, plus they understand how you feel as a student. Use your peers to discuss issues about practice and what resources they have used to help them.

Reflecting in and on practice

Most universities will expect you to keep a reflective diary. One of the most important things about reflecting on practice is doing it as soon as possible after the event. This may be in a discussion with your mentor, another member of staff or even a peer or writing it down in your diary for discussion later.

Students often say they cannot find anything to reflect on. That is impossible unless they have been asleep the whole time on placement! While dramatic events may seem more interesting to reflect on, you can learn just as much, if not more, by reflecting [cut] simple things. For instance, reflecting on helping a person to wash offers a whole range [cut] things you can learn from. What could you tell about the patient's physical condition, th[cut] nutritional and hydration status, their pain management? How could you tell this? What d[cut] you get to know about the person? How easy was it to talk to them? How were they feelin[cut] How did you know that? Did you make a difference to them? How did you know that?

So try to consider anything that is new or unfamiliar to you and also be aware to thi[cut] about things that went well, in addition to those things that did not go so well.

Self-Assessment

All nurses and midwives are expected to be lifelong learners, which means you nee[cut] to be able to assess your own knowledge and performance in order to identify yo[cut] developmental needs.

There may be a particular tool or framework that your university would like you to u[cut] in helping you to structure your self-assessment, but also use the criteria in your actio[cut] plan that you and your mentor have agreed that you will be judged upon. Look back [cut] Table 15.2. Can you answer yes to all the elements in all three columns? If yes then you ca[cut] probably assess yourself as competent in medicine administration, but you will obvious[cut] need to get this validated by your mentor.

As discussed in Chapter 14, feedback from others is a valuable way of getting a picture [cut] yourself and will help you in honing your skills of self-assessment. Ask for regular feedbac[cut] It is natural to be worried that you may not receive positive feedback and so not ask, b[cut] if there are areas you need to improve upon you need to know. Feedback that tells yo[cut] that you need to improve should be seen not as a criticism or a negative but as a mea[cut] for helping you to develop as a professional. If you are told you have areas you nee[cut] to improve upon ask for guidance on what you specifically need to do to demonstra[cut] improvement, this should be written up in your action plan.

Evaluating Practice Learning

On completion of your placement you will be required to evaluate both your own learnin[cut] and also your opinion of the placement area as a learning environment. This is an importan[cut] exercise as it gives feedback to the university and the placement itself about the quality of the area for learning. Improvements cannot be made if you don't give honest, constructive feedback. To help you evaluate your placement there is a useful checklist to be found in the Royal College of Nursing (RCN 2002) booklet *Helping Students Get the Best from Their Practice Placements. A Royal College of Nursing Toolkit.*

Conclusion

You must spend a minimum of 2300 hours in different placements during your pro-gramme – just think how much learning you can do in that time! To get the most from each placement you will need to be proactive in your learning. While your mentor will help facilitate your learning it is your responsibility to prepare, read, ask questions and get actively involved. More importantly enjoy yourself, your student days really are the best time in your life!

Tips

- Make contact with the placement before you start
- Do some pre-reading relevant to the area you are going to
- Arrive with an idea of what you want to learn and areas you need to improve upon
- Keep your eyes and ears open and ask to see and do things
- Get involved – it shows interest and motivation.
- Request feedback on a regular basis
- Evaluate your learning and the placement at the end.

Useful Websites

The Royal College of Nursing www.rcn.org.uk

The Nursing and Midwifery Council www.nmc-uk.org

Useful Publications Available via the Web

Nursing and Midwifery Council (NMC) (2002) *An NMC Guide for Students of Nursing and Midwifery.* Available at: www.nmc-uk.org/aFrameDisplay.aspx?DocumentID=1896

NMC (2004a) *The NMC Code of Professional Conduct: Standards for Conduct, Performan* *and Ethics.* London, NMC. Available at: www.nmc-uk.org/aFrameDisplay.asp: DocumentID=201

NMC (2004b) *Guidelines for the Administration of Medicines.* London, NMC. Available www.nmc-uk.org/aFrameDisplay.aspx?DocumentID=221

Royal College of Nursing (RCN) (2002) *Helping Students Get the Best from Their Pract* *Placements. A Royal College of Nursing Toolkit.* Available at: http://www.rcn.org.uk publications/pdf/helpingstudents.pdf

Royal College of Nursing (RCN) (2005) *Guidance for Mentors of Student Nurses and M.* *wives: an RCN Toolkit.* Available at: http://www.rcn.org.uk/publications/pd: guidance_for_ mentors.pdf

Chapter 16

Developing Your Clinical Skills

by Deann Cox and Steve Trenoweth

In this chapter you will learn about:

- **Your clinical role as a student**
- **The nature and range of clinical skills**
- **The complex interplay of various clinical skills**
- **How clinical skills must address biological, psychological and social needs**
- **Health and safety issues**
- **The role of clinical skills centres**
- **The importance of obtaining feedback on your clinical skills.**

Introduction

This chapter is not an instructional guide but an overview of how and why clinical skills are an important aspect of your nursing and midwifery practice. It is important to realize that you will need not only to perform a variety of skills in a competent manner, but that you must also practise safely. That is, you will need to demonstrate an ability to undertake tasks in an increasingly skilled, competent and confident manner and you must also appreciate the need for assessment of a range of risks relating to your clinical interventions.

This chapter focuses not only on the *doing* aspect of nursing and midwifery practice but also stresses the importance of *knowing* the rationale and evidence which underpins clinical intervention and also, importantly, why it is essential to consider the psychological and emotional impact that your clinical interventions may have on your patient group.

The Expectation of the Nursing/Midwifery Clinical Practice

Nurses and midwives practising in various contexts need to possess a wide range of skills, knowledge and values to underpin their clinical practice. The modern nurse/midwife will be expected to undertake a whole range of increasingly complex skills (such as prescribing certain medications, undertaking minor surgery, developing nurse-led services). The development of your clinical skills, however basic they may seem, is the starting point of this very important and exciting journey.

Your Clinical Role as a Student Nurse/Midwife

As a student nurse or midwife, you must remember that the regulations which apply to qualified nurses and midwives also apply to you. You are advised to read and understand the guidance and standards issued by the Nursing and Midwifery Council (NMC) which will not only highlight your role as a student in the clinical area, but will also state your responsibilities to your patients.

Furthermore, staff in clinical areas, including your mentor, will expect you to be able to practise safely and understand your limitations from the outset. You will also be expected to conduct yourself at all times in a professional manner. It is most likely that, initially, you will be observing the clinical practice of qualified and experienced nurses or midwives. It is important that you do not undertake any clinical interventions that you feel are beyond your level of ability. This is a key issue in safe practice and protecting the public. Remember throughout the development of your clinical skills you will be supervised by a qualified practitioner. However, if you feel that you are 'out of your depth' in your clinical practice, you must state this clearly and it is very important that you refrain from undertaking these duties.

What are Clinical Skills?

This may seem an obvious question. Clinical skills refer to those nursing or midwifery actions which enable you to carry out a healthcare related task and/or provide a service. However, it is important to clarify the complex and diverse range of clinical skills, which you need to practise safely within a modern healthcare context.

You may feel that you currently possess a number of skills that you use in everyday life which you may be able to apply to your clinical practice. However, in your clinical practice you will need to undertake a range of actions that are based on what is known to work best – and this includes *hand washing*! Therefore, you will be guided as to the most efficient and evidence based way to wash your hands so as to reduce the incidence of infection. The same principles will apply to a wide range of clinical skills – from the seemingly basic to the more complex.

Range and Extent of Clinical Skills

The range and extent of nursing and midwifery clinical skills is extraordinary. Here are just a few examples of the skills that you will need:

- Administration of medication via different routes
- Assessing the patient and making a nursing diagnosis
- Basic counselling/communication skills
- Basic observations (temperature, respiration, pulse, blood pressure)
- Care of the dying
- Collecting specimens and urinalysis
- Diet, nutrition and fluid intake
- Hygiene and hand decontamination

- Making beds
- Management of medication
- Moving and handling, including positioning the patient
- Pain assessment and management
- Promoting health
- Team working
- Using information technology in the clinical setting
- Wound care/management.

Additionally, there are some specialist skills that you will develop within your own special
Student midwives, for example, will learn about the palpation of the uterus; listening to
foetal heart using Pinard stethoscopes and foetal dopplers. Mental health nurses will le
counselling skills, how to de-escalate an angry or aggressive patient, and how to supp
a hallucinating patient.

Some of these can seem relatively straightforward – how complicated can it be to co
the number of times someone breathes per minute? However, this is in fact a very comp
task – for you are not only interested in the *rate* of respiration, but also whether or
someone seems in pain when they breath. Is there any noise, for example, associated w
their breathing? Is there a 'rattle' (suggestive of a build-up of fluid on the lungs or
infection) ? What is the *depth* and *pattern* of their breathing? Is it shallow? Is it regular?
the lungs inflate symmetrically? There are skills associated with noticing – picking up
subtle cues and clinical signs that would be missed by many people – and suggestive
increasing expertise in your practice.

So, what about making beds? (No doubt you noticed this in the above list!) This seems a v
trivial task – more associated with ritual and routine of a bygone age. Surely there are
clinical skills associated with making a bed! However, there are many issues associated w
making the less mobile patient, or those who are restricted to a bed, more comfortable.
example, you will need to consider the suitability and type of bed and mattress to prom
recovery and reduce the incidence of secondary problems, such as pressure sores. You
also need to consider your own health and safety here – if you are making a bed, can
height be adjusted? This is crucial to protect your spine! Furthermore, for the mental he
client who tends to neglect himself or herself, the act of encouraging and helping t
person to make their bed is an important contribution to developing their self-care ski

Surely washing your hands isn't a clinical skill? Do you really need to develop skills in h
to wash your hands? In your personal life you will have a view of standards of health

hygiene and you may feel that this is an area for which you need little or no guidance. However, the importance of understanding infection control and hygiene, and the skills of using the correct hand-washing technique, cannot be overemphasized. No doubt you have read about the concerns of increasing rate of methicillin resistant *Staphylococcus aureus* (MRSA) infections in hospitals. Effective and thorough hand decontamination is an important step to eradicating this within hospital environments (DoH 2004) which is, in reality, a complex and skilled activity quite unlike washing your hands at home.

The Interplay of Clinical Skills

It is important to realize that clinical skills are not simply about *doing*. That is, clinical skills are more than specific skilled nursing or midwifery actions but must include an awareness of why you are doing them and how this makes your clients feel. Let's take, as an example, wound care. In wound management, the development of your technical knowledge requires you to understand the nature of a wound, and concepts such as tissue viability. You will also need to be able to assess a wound accurately, giving detailed descriptions of your observations. This implies that you have developed the appropriate knowledge to notice those aspects of the wound, which are relevant or salient.

However, a skilled competent practitioner is also mindful of the need for infection control. This may involve taking the appropriate steps to protect themselves, and their patient, from cross contamination, such as effective hand washing and asepsis and the wearing of appropriate protective clothing. Furthermore, the skilled practitioner is aware of how distressing the injury might be for the patient, and ensures that they provide the appropriate reassurance. This requires a different set of clinical skills – psychological care skills – requiring the ability to empathize with the distressed patient and to use appropriate verbal and non-verbal communication in order to provide emotional support.

Lines of Demarcation

It has often been remarked that there are clear, but artificial, lines of demarcation in the clinical knowledge and skills used by those who predominately provide physical care, and those who predominantly provide psychological care. We say *artificial* because in reality nursing and midwifery care is said to be *holistic* (i.e. concerned with all aspects of the person). In providing holistic care, we see the person as having various needs – biological, psychological and social. Indeed, for ourselves as human beings it is natural for us to be aware of how our own physical health might affect how we feel emotionally, how we thi and how we behave. So, in terms of our clinical actions, we must be aware that the techni application of clinical skills (no matter how expert) is insufficient unless it considers, a responds to, the totality of the patient's experience including their psychological and soc needs. This requires a wide range of diverse clinical skills.

Sometimes, this line of demarcation is drawn by our own profession, sometimes by t services in which we work, sometimes by ourselves, but not necessarily by the nature our patients' needs. The danger is that we see people with physical health needs as havi no psychological or other needs; and people with mental health problems as having biological needs. Certainly, in the latter case, recent attention has been drawn to the ne to improve the physical wellbeing of, and nursing care that is given to, people with men health problems (DoH 2006).

Furthermore, in recent years there has been increasing evidence that social conte and psychological wellbeing are important issues in illness and recovery, which can influenced by our thoughts, beliefs, and emotions (Kleijnen 2005). In real terms, the drawing the line of demarcation between the biological, the psychological and the soc can affect the clinical outcomes of our patients.

Health and Safety

Health and safety practice is an essential clinical skill and it is crucial that you are mind of the various potential hazards arising from clinical environments. You will recei appropriate training during your programme in order to be able to respond effectively such hazards, so as to facilitate your own health and safety and that of colleagues, a ensure your patients and members of the public are safe. You must attend such traini and ensure that the skills you are taught are rehearsed until they become a routine part your clinical practice.

While it is beyond the scope of this chapter to give you an in-depth overview of all t health and safety issues relating to clinical practice, there are a number of issues that ne highlighting.

One of the most common reasons for sickness in the health service is musculoskele and back injuries. It is of vital importance that you are able to undertake the necessa assessments, and are skilled in the use of correct moving and handling techniques prevent back injuries. In clinical practice, you might be tempted to cut corners, especially if the clinical area is busy, but *do not under any circumstances deviate from the training*. Damage to your spine can be devastating and have profound implications for your personal life and your career. You will find that there will be regular manual handling updates offered by your university and this is to ensure that you are appraised of any possible changing guidance and legal frameworks. While you must always follow advice given to you by the university, there are useful information leaflets available on manual handling at the Health and Safety Executive's website (www.hse.gov.uk/pubns/manlinde.htm).

There are many other health and safety issues of which you need to be mindful. In recent years, there have been concerns in relation to blood borne infections, and the administration of injections and safe disposal of associated materials (such as needles and other contaminated items) is vital to ensure your own health and safety (and that of others). Additionally, the Health and Safety Executive singles out the following as being particularly common: slips and trips from spilled liquids or other hazards; dermatitis and allergic reactions, including latex allergies; stress; and assaults and violence. Each university and clinical service will have polices and procedures in place to manage these risks which you must be aware of. Further reading materials on these issues, and useful websites, can be found at the end of this chapter.

The overarching clinical skill here is to be watchful and mindful of potential risks associated within healthcare environments and to ensure that you take appropriate steps to manage and reduce such hazards.

The Role of the Clinical Skills Centre

Each university will have a venue where you will be able to develop your clinical skills. Such clinical skills centres provide an environment that mimics the clinical area. Skills sessions will be timetabled throughout your programme, and will be relevant to your learning outcomes and development.

The key emphasis of clinical skills centres is to offer you a safe environment for the rehearsal of the practice of nursing and midwifery, often working in small groups, which allows close supervision, support and development of your skills. In addition to the demonstration of a wide variety of clinical skills, you will be taught underpinning anatomy and physiology followed by supervised repetition of the skill. You will be expected to work closely with your student colleagues where you will have opportunities to share your learning and experiences.

Simulation of the clinical environment has been possible for a number of years. You cou be asked to 'role play' – a useful technique in helping you to develop an understandi of what the patient or relative experiences. Some skills centres employ actors as patie who are given clear and detailed roles to play or have high fidelity manikins which respo to interventions, such as Meti Man (Medical Education Technologies Inc.). You might a find that the role play scenario makes realistic demands by reproducing ward noises, a realistic interruptions, while you are trying to concentrate on providing care. This is r meant to confuse you but to orientate you to the real life complexity of clinical worki and decision making.

Assessment Feedback

Your performance in undertaking a particular clinical skill might be video or audio tap This allows you to see first hand areas where you performed well and where you requ development. It is also important that you obtain tutor/facilitator feedback and clarificati of points or issues which seem unclear. Remember that clinical skills development is incremental and cumulative process – one skill often builds on another. This means tha you are unsure of a particular skill then you have a rocky foundation upon which to bu others. Ask the tutor to demonstrate to you how it should be done, watch them clos and then ask them to watch you undertaking the task. Don't forget to ask them if you ha got it right!

How will you know when you are competent? Well, this is a skill in itself and relates to yo ability for self-monitoring and self-awareness, recognizing that what you are doing is b for the patient, based on evidence, and what is safest for you and your colleagues.

Finally, the motivation to develop and improve on your clinical skills here must come fro you. You should allow yourself as many opportunities to rehearse and repeat the skill necessary until you feel proficient; this allows you to learn at your own level and spe while always considering patient safety as your priority.

Tips

- In the clinical skills sessions, remember to wear clothes that are suitable, such as loos fitting trousers, tee-shirts and flat, securely fastened shoes (Some centres may well exp you to wear your uniform)

- Practise and rehearse clinical skills regularly
- Ensure that you attend any planned clinical skills update
- Remember: clinical skills allow you to respond effectively to the biological, psychological and social needs of your patients.

References

Department of Health (DoH) (2004) *Towards Cleaner Hospitals and Lower Rates of Infection.* London, DoH.
   Available at: www.dh.gov.uk/assetRoot/04/08/58/61/04085861.pdf
Department of Health (DoH) (2006) *From Values to Action: The Chief Nursing Officer's Review of Mental Health Nursing.* London, DoH.
   Available at: www.dh.gov.uk/assetRoot/04/13/38/40/04133840.pdf
Kleijnen, J. (2005) How important is the biopsychosocial approach? Some examples from research. In White, P. (ed) *Biopsychosocial Medicine: an Integrated Approach to Understanding Illness.* Oxford, Oxford University Press.

Further Reading

Al-Damouk, M., Pudney, E. and Bleetman, A. (2004) Hand hygiene and aseptic technique in the emergency department. *J Hosp Infect.*, 56(2), 137–41
Health and Safety Executive (2002) *Interventions to Control Stress at Work in Hospital Staff.* Norwich, HSE Books/HMSO.
   Available at: www.hse.gov.uk/research/crr_pdf/2002/crr02435.pdf
McCabe, C. and Timmins, F. (2006) *Communication Skills for Nursing Practice.* Basingstoke, Palgrave.
Peate, I. (2005) *Compendium of Clinical Skills for Student Nurses.* Chichester, Wiley.

Useful Websites

Health and Safety Executive: www.hse.gov.uk/healthservices/index.htm
Latex Allergy Support Group: www.lasg.co.uk

Section **4**

Survival Skills

In this section, the authors help you to consider some of the challenges within the programme and offer tips and advice on how to respond effectively.

This section will enable you to consider how you might marshal resources to cope with some of the personal and professional challenges arising from the programme. Students often remark on how anxiety provoking examinations can be and working with new colleagues in busy healthcare environments can also be stressful. This section will help you to develop coping strategies and to consider who might be best placed to assist you with this process.

Chapter 17

Surviving the Clinical Environment

by Kris Ramgoolam, Stella Brophy, Eddie Meyler and Steve Trenoweth

This chapter will consider the following:

- **The importance of developing self-awareness as a survival mechanism**
- **Why resisting the pressure to conform is important**
- **How to establish professional boundaries and productive working relationships**
- **Understanding power relationships**
- **The importance of managing stress**
- **Preparing to move on.**

Introduction

Clinical practice can be very emotionally challenging. You will experience more during y
nursing/midwifery education than many people see in their lifetime! You will see a num
of different life events, from birth to death, from someone receiving a diagnosis of seri
illness to someone being told that their cancer has responded successfully to treatme
There will be some highs and some lows. The experience of practice will inevitably pror
you to ask questions regarding the meaning of health and illness.

When you see children diagnosed with cancer, people with profound disabilities,
self-harming young person, you will be expected to provide care while putting your o
personal feelings and values to one side. This can be difficult, but being able to deal w
the emotional impact of clinical practice is necessary for your personal and professio
development as a nurse or midwife. So, what do you need to do to be able to surv
emotionally in the clinical setting?

Developing Self-Awareness

Survival in clinical practice is facilitated by a personal honesty and openness. You
need to develop a frank awareness of your 'self' and be able to ask searching questi
of yourself and others around you. You will certainly need to consider what annoys y
what upsets you and what makes you angry. Sometimes, we may lack awareness as to v
we have acted in a particular way. We may be the type of person that takes on too m
challenges, finding it difficult to say no to people. We may also spend time trying to ple
and appease others. We may strive for perfection in what we do and fear failure.

It is an essential requirement for surviving the clinical setting to think about who you
as a person, and what underlies your behaviour in different situations. This requires y
to be honest with yourself and accept your limitations while you are learning new sk
It will be helpful to reflect upon well-intentioned comments from your mentor and ot
members of the care team. This will help you to understand your emotional response
challenging situations.

A lack of self-awareness can have a profound impact on your personal and professic
development. Being honest with yourself can be anxiety provoking, however. You will na
rally have a self-concept, that is, an idea of who you are, what you are good at, and what y

are not so good at. But in nursing and midwifery you are likely to receive feedback from other people, who may have different ideas regarding your skills, abilities and knowledge. This may be a new and difficult experience for you. You may feel vulnerable and exposed at times.

It is not uncommon for people to come into nursing/midwifery having had personal painful experiences of their own, such as miscarriages, divorces, bereavements or illness. This can be a positive advantage in healthcare practice, as it promotes understanding of human suffering and facilitates empathy. However, there is a danger that if these experiences have not been satisfactorily resolved then the emotional pain may remain.

It is understandable, therefore, that some people 'survive' painful experiences by closing themselves off emotionally, becoming detached from other people. For the nurse/midwife this is problematic for many reasons. Avoidance is not a satisfactory long-term coping mechanism, but a way of containing personal anxiety in the short term. This can limit your personal and professional development by reducing your ability to empathize with others or take on board new ideas. If we are defensive, then we may become angry in the face of perceived personal criticism. We may be in denial of our personal developmental needs, such as a lack of clinical knowledge or skills. We may lack an awareness of the complex dynamics of interpersonal situations – and have a limited understanding of, or concern for, others' points of view. We may blame others unfairly for problems in the clinical area. We may become cynical. The problem with this is that one's personal emotional survival is seen to be more important than the survival of the patient and clinical team. Understanding and resolving such defensive behaviour is essential for survival in the clinical setting.

Resisting the Pressure to Conform

The establishment of positive, professional relationships is important in surviving the clinical environment. Professional relationships are built on shared and agreed expectations of each other. You may on occasions find yourself being pressurized into blindly adopting the rules and practices of the clinical environment. In order to survive you may feel the pressure to conform, to acquire the norms and values of the practice setting, however inappropriate they may seem. It is the mark of a professional to challenge, and ask searching question with the aim of improving practice and patient care. But this can also bring with it tensions and anxieties.

Questioning existing practices requires the skills of assertion. Technically, being assertive is the ability to state your case, clearly and firmly, but not confrontationally or aggressively.

However, while an assertive person appreciates, respects and understands others' vie points, they may not feel able to agree. Assertive people also tend to have confide in their own personal and professional core values and beliefs. This means that asser people are able to resist the pressure to conform blindly. They are, in fact, their own pers and are better placed to cope with the complex personal demands of surviving clin environments and of providing care which is based on sound evidence rather than rit and routine.

Establishing Professional Boundaries

It is often commented upon by students that a good relationship with their mentor see to be the lynchpin between their success and failure in the clinical environment. In f in order to survive it is essential to foster and develop a positive, professional relations with your mentor, with clear expectations and boundaries, from the outset.

Similarly, developing and establishing professional relationships with patients and ot members of the professional team can facilitate your survival and the emotional clim of your clinical placement can be crucial to your learning. As a new member of team you should feel psychologically safe to ask questions, or highlight issues of conc without the fear of intimidation and alienation or fear that the outcome of your clin practice assessment will be compromised. If you are unable to express your view: a safe environment, you will miss opportunities to learn and you may be unwilling communicate your developmental needs.

A survival strategy often adopted by student nurses and midwives within clinical envir ments is that of making friends, and socializing, with members of the professional te and patients. You might also feel that you should self-disclose personal information, s as family issues, or you may share anecdotes regarding your personal life. Be careful to overstep professional boundaries as you may experience a sense of vulnerability in practice placement if you divulge too much sensitive personal information.

However, at times such informality can be positive, and can facilitate a more o discussion of sensitive issues within the clinical area. You might be more inclined to sh your hopes and fears with those you feel more comfortable with. However, this a has inherent dangers if not handled well, as there might be a blurring of personal a professional boundaries. That is, you may lose sight of your role as a learner, and not able to differentiate the personal from the professional aspects of relationships. This mi mean that, for example, feedback on your professional knowledge and skills may be seen as a criticism of you as a person, or a patient may misinterpret your professional behaviour as a developing personal relationship.

So, while establishing positive, professional working relationship with others in the clinical environment is important to your survival, you must be mindful of establishing and maintaining appropriate boundaries with colleagues and patients. If you feel that you are unable to express your needs within the professional team, then you should discuss this with your mentor, ward manager or representative from the university. You may also feel the need to make a complaint. Whatever you feel you need to do, if you have maintained clear professional boundaries, your actions will not be seen by others in personal terms.

Understanding Power Relationships

Professional relationships are marked by boundaries that regulate the way in which colleagues relate to each other. Relationships can initially seem very formalized with people addressing each other using formal titles, such as 'Sister' or 'Staff Nurse'. As a student you will need to appreciate that this level of formality is often a way of creating order that can have both positive and negative implications for the delivery of care.

A professional team is often hierarchical, and is by its very nature characterized by differential power relationships. Someone is 'in charge', someone is the 'manager' and so on. This is usually a natural and efficient way of organizing teams of people. However, you might need to consider your capacity for acting on instructions, being delegated to, or indeed, accepting critical comments about your professional performance. If you are a mature student, for example, you might be taking instructions from someone who is considerably younger than you, and this might pose problems for you. This is an issue that you may need to reflect upon in relation to your role as a potential employee and team member. To survive in clinical environments it is necessary for you to understand and accept the hierarchical nature of working in teams as an occupational fact of life.

A subtle way of maintaining power relationships is the symbolic use of jargon, abbreviations and terminology, which can be very confusing to the outsider. This might be seen as a way of gatekeeping professional knowledge, and of excluding outsiders, and you may feel intimidated by this form of communication. Good communication and understanding of professional language is essential to learning and promoting safe care. Mistakes can be made through assumptions and a general lack of understanding. In order to survive in

clinical environments, it is important that you should not feel intimidated by the seemin
esoteric use of language and symbols in healthcare practice. To ensure a positive learn
experience in the clinical environment, you should never be afraid of seeking clarificat
and asking questions.

As a student, you should be perceived as a member of the care team. Indeed, you r
want to be perceived as such. However, you may also feel under pressure to perfc
certain clinical skills without appropriate or adequate supervision, especially if you
working in a busy clinical environment. As a consequence, you may find yourself i
situation where you are asked to do something that you are not sure of. Never be afr
to say 'I don't know how to do this'. The focus of your time in the clinical environm
is on your learning and development – remember your 'supernumerary status'! It is
strength of a mature and professional approach to clinical learning to declare when
do not know how to perform a particular procedure, and remember never to go bey
your depth.

Managing Stress

Stress is, it seems, an inevitable fact of life! We all feel stressed from time to time.
not unusual, abnormal or a sign of weakness. Indeed, a certain amount of stress is hel
to us – it acts as a spur to action. However, when we have too much stress in our li
or we experience stress that we are unable to satisfactorily respond to, we may becc
'distressed'.

Identifying and managing unacceptable levels of personal stress is a necessary aspec
surviving clinical practice. Sometimes stress can arise from our day-to-day lives. Sometir
there may be additional strain placed upon us from particular stressors or life eve
such as money worries, or concerns over the health of a family member. Certainly, th
may be stressors that arise from clinical practice, such as conflicts with another per
in the team or the challenge of providing care to people with multiple or serious ne
As a student, your programme may also place upon you certain demands that may v
add to your stress levels, such as trying to meet deadlines for the submission of y
assessments.

Everyone copes with stress in their own way. Some people like to develop a clear
focused strategy to confront stressors directly. Sometimes, however, the stressed/distres
person may not be aware of how stressed they are, or what the source of their stress mi

be. Sometimes, a person might lack an ability to take effective action to reduce stress. Here, the stressed person may resort to unhealthy ways of coping, such as avoidance behaviour or resorting to drugs or alcohol, which not only do not resolve the original stressor but can add a whole host of secondary problems.

It is important to adopt a healthy approach to managing stress and not to let things build up. If you are feeling stressed, then acknowledge this and try not to feel embarrassed. If you feel that you need some assistance, there are many people involved with your programme that can help you to manage stress or who can offer a sympathetic ear. Discuss it with a trusted friend or approach your mentor, programme leader or personal tutor. Don't forget that every university will have its own free and confidential student counselling service and you may feel it appropriate, or indeed prefer, to offload or discuss issues with someone unconnected to your programme.

Terminating Relationships

Moving on is a necessary and inevitable part of being a student. You start your clinical placement in the full knowledge that your experience there is time limited. This can be reassuring if you are not enjoying your placement, but if your experience there is a positive one, you may not want to leave! Moving on, therefore, can be for a variety of reasons an emotional experience. For example, if you have been working closely with very ill clients whose prognosis is poor and with whom you have established a close professional relationship, you might feel reluctant to go. But go you must in order to progress through your programme.

It is important, in survival terms, to have a sense of closure when you are completing a clinical practice experience. You should be mindful that nursing and midwifery care is a very human experience, and you must be aware of the possible impact that your departure may have on your patients, and the clinical team. At the end of the practice it is important to inform patients that you have worked with closely that you are leaving the clinical area, and to have the opportunity to say goodbye. Terminating relationships appropriately with team members is equally important.

For yourself, the end of the placement may be a time for considerable reflection. You will need to take stock of, and reflect upon, the placement so that you may put into perspective your experiences and how much you have learnt. Your future survival is facilitated by being realistic about your ongoing personal and professional developmental needs.

Tips

- Be honest with yourself – consider your abilities and developmental needs
- Listen and appreciate constructive feedback from others
- Be assertive and try to resist the pressure to conform blindly
- Take time to consider and develop professional working relationships in the pract setting
- Invest time in developing your relationship with your mentor
- Understand the hierarchical nature of clinical teams
- Maintain contact with your university if you feel your concerns are not being ackno edged in clinical practice
- Recognize and respond to challenges to your emotional well being.

Chapter 18

How to Survive Exams

by Ian Chisholm-Bunting and Sue Vernon

This chapter looks at:

- **Planning and managing your revision**
- **Identifying and using your preferred learning style to memorise information for examinations**
- **Answering exam questions**
- **Managing the actual examination**
- **Tackling stress.**

Introduction

> We are what we repeatedly do. Excellence, then, is not an act, but a habit
>
> Aristotle

Examinations, perhaps more than anything else in education, can cause anxiety. Howe
in this chapter we will show you that much of this anxiety is unwarranted, and v
preparation you will develop the skills to succeed in your exams.

Passing an exam means some hard work, good organizational skills and being sure of w
you have to do. So, surviving, and being successful in, your exams, is not only about w
you know but how well prepared you are.

Planning and Managing Your Revision

Managing your time

A theme which emerges throughout this book is being proactive in your learnin
planning, thinking ahead and managing yourself and your time. This is particularly true
examinations. Whatever you do, do not leave your preparations for examinations until
last minute! There are also many personal demands on us but it is very important to m
sure you find time to revise. We suggest that you use the revision timetable (Table 18.1
plan your time. For each week of revision left before the exam, we suggest you:

1. Fill in everything you *have* to do on the revision timetable – this includes your univer
   work and personal responsibilities. Make sure you know exactly what topics you n
   to prepare for the exam and then plan your revision, allowing enough time for all top
2. Break down your study into short periods; most people find that 45 minutes to an h
   and half in length is ideal. However, vary this if it suits your study habits. Decide wh
   you work best – are you a 'night owl' (someone who likes to work late into the night
   are you an 'early bird' (someone who likes to get up and work very early)?
3. Plan regular breaks between your studies and ensure you have regular nutritious me
   and drinks as this will keep your energy levels up.
4. Set aside a revision area and ask your flatmates/family to respect this space! If i
   difficult to work at home, go to your university or local library or team up with a frie
5. Make sure you stick to this timetable! Pin it up at home or put it in your revision file
   that you can remind yourself of the schedule you have set yourself.

Table 18.1 Revision timetable

	Week beginning					Exam date	
	Monday	Tuesday	Wednesday	Thursday	Friday	Saturday	Sunday
6.00 a.m.							
7.00 a.m.							
8.00 a.m.							
9.00 a.m.							
10.00 a.m.							
11.00 a.m.							
12.00 a.m.							
1.00 p.m.							
2.00 p.m.							
3.00 p.m.							
4.00 p.m.							
5.00 p.m.							
6.00 p.m.							
7.00 p.m.							
8.00 p.m.							
9.00 p.m.							
10.00 p.m.							
11.00 p.m.							
12.00 p.m.							

Collecting information

It is also important that you collect relevant information for each topic you are revising. Make a careful decision on the number of topics you need to revise so that you are confident you know enough for the exam. A broad guide to relevant information can be found in your Module and Programme handbooks (and in particular the essential and further reading lists). We suggest that you also pay particular attention to the Learning Outcomes for your module and programme as these are the criteria you will need to meet in order to complete a course.

It is a good idea to collect everything together for each revision topic in one folder. Make photocopies where you can, so that you can use highlighters to identify important information. If you can get hold of old exam papers, use these to give you an idea of the types of question which are asked and to check that the format hasn't changed. If no previous exam papers are available, ask your lecturer to provide you with a specimen exam paper.

Once you have collected sources from which to revise, make sure you are actively involved in your revision by writing notes on relevant information. When you are taking notes, we

suggest that you leave plenty of space on the page, so that you can add further informat
if necessary. If you have a visual memory, use coloured pens, highlighters, bullet poi
arrows and so on, in order to highlight key points.

Memorizing Information

Summarizing and remembering information

Once you are happy that you have taken enough notes on each topic, you will need
summarize these, so that you can start the process of memorizing information. Write
points on index cards and group them by topic. Keep these with you at all times, so t
you can read them repeatedly and then test yourself to see whether you can recall
information. Ask family and friends to test you and practise until you are word perfect!

Identifying your preferred learning style

We don't all learn in the same way and tend to adopt styles with which we feel m
comfortable. If you can identify your preferred learning style, not only will it help y
general learning, it will help you to remember information. For example, if you are a vis
learner, you will remember things as an image; if you are an auditory learner, you
remember sounds, for example, voices, discussions; if you are a kinaesthetic learner, y
will use both of the above and will enjoy being physically involved in your learning.

Complete the questionnaire (Table 18.2) in order to find out what kind of learner you a

Look for your highest score as this will indicate your preferred learning style. You n
find that you have one score that is much higher than any of the others. This shows y
preferred learning style. Alternatively, you might have two scores which are similar. T
means that you use both styles equally well. If all three scores are similar, again you ha
no particular preference and use all learning styles. Obviously, the more learning styles y
can use, the better your learning will be in different situations.

Memory techniques using your learning style(s)

The following table will give you some ideas for using each of the learning styles in relat
to revision and using your memory effectively.

Table 18.2   Learning styles questionnaire

Read the following questions and ring the letter at the left hand side to indicate which answer you feel is most appropriate. Only ring one answer.

To remind you of the types of learning styles, look at the following key:
V = Visual learner (learns by seeing)
A = Auditory learner (learns by hearing)
K = Kinaesthetic learner (learns by being actively involved)

When you spell, do you
    V   see the word?
    A   sound the word out?
    K   write the word down and make sure it feels right?

When you remember specific incidents, do you
    V   see well focused, colour pictures?
    A   hear sounds?
    K   see a few pictures with movement in them?

When you are thinking really hard and concentrating, are you distracted by
    V   untidiness?
    A   noise?
    K   movement?

When you are angry, do you
    V   silently seethe inside?
    A   shout and scream?
    K   clench your fists, grit your teeth, stomp about and go away angry?

When you forget someone or something, do you
    V   forget names but remember faces?
    A   forget faces but remember names?
    K   remember best where, when and what you did?

When you are reading, do you
    V   enjoy reading description and make your own picture?
    A   hear the characters talking?
    K   like to act it out?

When you are relaxing, do you
    V   watch TV, read, see a play?
    A   listen to music, the radio?
    K   play sports or games?

When you are learning, do you prefer
    V   work that is written and drawn in many colours?
    A   to listen to a lecture or be told instructions?
    K   to participate in activities, making or doing?

(Continues)

Table 18.2   (*continued*)

When you are talking, do you
    V   talk little and are reluctant to listen for too long?
    A   like to listen and want to talk as well?
    K   talk with your hands and gesture a lot?

When you are being rewarded or praised by someone, do you prefer to
    V   receive a written note?
    A   hear it said to you?
    K   be given a pat on the back or a hug?

Now add up the number of answers for which you circled V, A and K.
Total number of V's =
Total number of A's =
Total number of K's =

A visual learner learns best by seeing things. So you could:

- Use colours, patterns and pictures to help fix and remember a 'picture of information' your mind. For example, you could draw a hand and associate five key points with i use a clock face or a tree with branches each of which means something to you
- Photocopy reading material and, using different colours, highlight particular pieces information – remember the information by recalling the colour
- Use spider diagrams to recall information and plan answers to questions
- Recall a visual demonstration of a skill and 'replay' this through in your mind, so that y can write down the details easily
- Watch your peers/tutors practising clinical skills.

An auditory learner learns best by listening to information. So you could:

- Record all lectures and seminars (only with your lecturer's permission); play these b and make notes on information particularly related to your revision topics. Better sti you use a digital recorder you can upload the material on to your computer and forr your notes in a style which suits your learning
- Recall a seminar or class discussion on a particular topic and record important po raised, uploading these again on to your computer if using a digital recorder
- Discuss important points with friends.

A kinaesthetic learner learns best by using a combination of methods and be actively involved in learning. So you could:

• Use a combination of all of the above and when practising clinical skills assessments, talk through each step, which will help your brain to remember the sequence of actions.

Answering Exam Questions

Answer the question, the whole question and nothing but the question!

The most important aspect of sitting any written exam is to *answer* the question you have been asked! This does not mean writing all you know about a topic, but focusing on the question and writing a structured answer in whatever format is required, for example report, essay, short answer.

In order to understand the question correctly you need to identify:

• The main focus of the question
• The instruction words. These tell you *what* you have to do with the material, for example discuss, evaluate, compare and contrast
• Any other important words. These could be words that need defining or limit the scope of the question in some way
• How many parts there are to the question. You could be asked to do two things, for example outline and critically evaluate. . . or identify and discuss. . ..

Underline important words and different parts of the question, as this will make planning your answer much easier. Have a look at the following question to see how this technique has been applied.

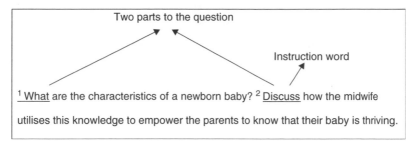

Planning your answer

If you are taking any kind of written unseen exam, it is essential to make some sort of plan *before you start writing.*

You could:

- Put your ideas down in a spider diagram and then number these in order of importan
- Make a list of key points and organize them into paragraphs, with the first sentence
  each paragraph as the key point
- Jot down any references beside these points.

Remember that you haven't got a lot of time, so select the information that directly answ
the question. Do not waste words on providing unnecessary background information –
right to the point.

Useful strategies for different types of exams

Unseen exams

For unseen exams that require an essay, report or short answer format, try to ensure t
you revise more topics than the number of questions you have to answer. This will ens
that you have additional information, in case you don't like the look of one of the questio
Make sure you analyse the question carefully, so that you use only the information t
answers the question!

Try to remember the surname(s) and date of publication of the sources you have use
your revision and insert these, where appropriate. If you are asked to bring in a pre-prepa
list of references, make sure you have not made any other notes on this.

Some university programmes use scenarios in unseen exams. These are passages of t
describing a set of events normally related to a disease process or the management
patient. Here we suggest that you familiarize yourself with the scenario, read and re-r
the scenario. Highlight or underline facts and key words. Read and re-read the questio
to make sure you understand what is required. It would be a good idea to produce a spi
diagram to answer the question(s); make sure your plan answers the question.

Ensure that you refer to the scenario and the question throughout the essay, use te
such as 'from the scenario' or 'the scenario describes' and 'the scenario states'. Finally, m
sure you use your wider reading to give your answer depth and show detailed knowle
of issues.

Seen exams

You might be given a seen exam question, well in advance of an exam. You are then expected to develop your knowledge of the topic and answer the question as fully as possible. Therefore, when you take the exam, you are writing a prepared and rehearsed essay on the topic.

Once you have completed all your research, produce a plan that answers the question. If you can, discuss this plan with your lecturer before you write a draft answer. Write a draft answer and again, if you can, discuss this with your lecturer. Make any necessary changes and produce another draft. When you are happy with your essay, practise writing it to see how long it takes. If it takes longer than the time you will have in your exam, try to shorten it, by deleting irrelevant information.

You will probably not be able to remember your essay word for word, but using your preferred learning style, memorize your plan, so that you can reproduce your essay in the examination room. You will be expected to refer to sources accurately, giving authors' names and date(s) of publication, so again use a method which suits you, to remember these.

You might be given a scenario well ahead of the exam, but will usually not know the questions. Here we suggest that you highlight all the issues that the scenario raises and think of questions that these may raise. Use the learning outcomes for this part of your programme which might help you to identify the kinds of questions that may be asked in the exam.

Make sure you read widely around the issues identified in the scenario. Ask whether your lecturer is willing to have a general class discussion on the scenario. You might like to work with other students, in order to identify all the issues raised in the scenario.

Multiple Choice Questionnaires (MCQs)

Generally, you are given a set of questions, with several possible answers; you have to identify the correct answer. We suggest that you revise the subject(s) covered by the multiple choice questionnaires (MCQs). Many students take a gambler's chance that one in three of the answers is correct and thus seem to believe that this type of exam is about guesswork. While this type of approach plays a part, it is no substitute for knowing yo subject!

Some answers you may know immediately to be wrong, so exclude the wrong answe and concentrate on the potential correct answers. Review the question again, choose yo answer and move on. If you are unsure of an answer, highlight or mark the question ar return to the question at the end of the exam. You might then find that you have a clea idea of the correct answer. If you have no idea of the answer, just choosing one is bett than leaving a blank.

Try to use your time wisely in the exam. Answer the questions to which you know th answer first and then spend time on analysis of problematic questions. You may find th you know more than you first thought! Once you have completed your answers che your paper to ensure you have marked your chosen answers in the correct order. Mar students lose marks by being careless with regard to time management.

Objective Structured Clinical Examinations (OSCEs)

This means you have to demonstrate clinical skills in front of others who will be assessir you on the basis of your skills performance. Universities assess objective structure clinical examinations (OSCEs) in many ways. Some may audio or video record the skil demonstration and the student is then given a pass or fail grade. Other institutions us a skills laboratory to simulate clinical environments and student performance is assesse within them or through virtual learning computer programs. Finally, some universitie assess in the clinical environment itself, using actors or volunteer clients. Regardless setting, your clinical skills are being tested.

Being observed makes people nervous – it is a fact of life! Practise your clinical skill a often as you can until it becomes natural to you. Do this also in front of family, friends colleagues. You may not always have the equipment, but talk through the skill in front an audience and ask for feedback. This will get you used to performing in front of others

If you make a mistake in your skill examination, immediately acknowledge you have mad an error and correct it. Such acknowledgement means you have recognized the situatio and dealt with it. This could mean the difference between a pass and a fail grade. Finall you may be asked to comment or reflect on your performance. If you haven't done s already, acknowledge anything that you know went wrong and say what you should hav done.

Managing the Actual Examination

Try to find out as much as you can about the exam beforehand. For example, when, where and at what time is the exam? What is the format of the exam? Is it the same as in previous years? What learning outcomes does the exam assess? How are the marks distributed between questions? If you have a temporary or permanent physical or unseen disability or a specific learning difficulty, it is also important to contact the appropriate department at your university as soon as possible, to check that special arrangements have been put in place.

So that you arrive feeling fully prepared and calm on the day of the examination, make sure you have everything ready the night before. Remind yourself of the time and place of the exam and think about your journey. Collect together all the equipment you might need, such as:

- Pens, pencils, rubber, ruler
- Calculator – assuming that you have been given clear permission to use them
- List of references (if required)
- Energy sweets – these are useful in providing glucose which your body can use in quick bursts to power your brain cells.
- Water – again, your brain needs this to function properly
- A lucky mascot!

On the day of the exam, try to avoid groups of students who are talking to each other and clearly making each other nervous. Go into the exam room in plenty of time to settle down and, if necessary, practise some slow deep breathing or relaxation techniques to focus your attention. It is important that you arrive on time as it is common practice for university regulations not to allow students into the examination hall once the exam has started.

The start of the exam

Listen carefully to the invigilator's instructions. Then, ensure that you fully read the whole exam paper through including the instructions. In unseen exams, decide in which order you are going to tackle the questions. Think about whether you want to tackle the question you feel most confident about first of all. Doing this can give you confidence. Alternatively, you might want to tackle a more difficult question first, while you are still fresh.

Don't worry if other people seem to start writing furiously around you. Making sure you understand the question, thinking and planning your answer is a vital part of taking exams and you need to allow time for this. If your exam requires a lengthy answer to a question it is common practice to start each answer on a new page. This will allow you to add more information at the bottom of an answer, if you find you have left something out.

Managing your time

It is important to manage your time carefully, so that you answer all of the required questions. You might find that some questions carry more marks than others. If this is the case, you should spend more time on these. You must also make sure you attempt each question, in order to have a chance of getting the maximum number of marks for the exam.

Have a look at the following example showing how a student has decided to use her time. You can see that she has allowed 55 minutes per question, so that she has ten minutes left over. This is so she can read through the paper at the beginning and check that everything is in order at the end.

How long is the exam?
Two hours (120 minutes)
How many questions will I have to answer?
Two questions – one from each section of the paper
How much time will I have for each question?
One hour (60 minutes)
How will I use the time for each question?
Understanding and thinking about the question five minutes
Planning five minutes
Writing 40 minutes
Checking five minutes
Total time: 55 minutes

In order to keep to the time schedule you have set yourself, you might find it useful to take your watch off and put it on your desk so that you can watch the time carefully. You could also bring in a small, but silent clock.

One of the ways to avoid time management problems is to practise planning and writing timed answers to questions at home. You will then know how much you can write in a specific time and how your hand stands up to writing continuously!

What to do if time runs out

If you run out of time, you can implement the following emergency action. However, you must always check that these strategies are acceptable at your university. We would suggest the following emergency action:

* If you have spent too long on the previous question(s), try to make up time on the next question(s)
* Complete unfinished questions in note form
* Plan a whole answer in note form, but make sure it is legible
* At the end of an unfinished answer, refer the marker back to your plan (this is just one of the reasons to complete a plan).

At the end of the exam

Listen carefully to the invigilator's instructions. Check through your paper – it's better to have a last minute inspiration, rather than remembering something on the way home!

Look for:

* Words missed out
* Spelling mistakes – particularly in anatomy and physiology
* Incorrect dates and names.

Resist the temptation to hang around to discuss what you did or didn't do with your colleagues. This may be demoralising and depressing. You've done all you can, so forget the exam, and take a break.

Tackling Stress

Mention the word exam and many students immediately associate it with stress! Exams are designed to put the student under pressure and call for different skills compared with course work. Try to differentiate between *stress* (which can be positive and thus improve performance) and *distress* (which is negative and harmful to performance). Do not to allow yourself to become distressed by an exam.

Manage your stress by managing yourself. Recognize that revising for your exam will cause stress; see the stress as positive and useful to you in terms of preparing you for the

challenge of the exam. Use stress to improve your performance. Start by revising for h
an hour and increase this time bit by bit. As you achieve a new milestone, reward yours
with a treat! Think of a reward for when your exams are over. It may be something
complex as a holiday, or as simple as a body massage. The reward should be personal
you; it has to be your idea or it will have little value to you. Think of this reward every tir
you find yourself getting distressed because it all seems too hard or you are becomi
demoralized.

Being in control of your revision will mean you will feel less stressed. Organize your revisi
using a revision planner and manage your time on a daily basis. Much of how we proce
information is linked to repetition; think about what kind of learner you are and choc
the best revision process. Others may give you guidance, but remember everyone v
have their own method of revising and, providing yours works, stick to it. If you find it is
working, then try another strategy. Don't give up!

Maintain regular exercise during revision; fit it into your schedule as it is very help
in relieving distress and nervous tension. If you can, plan at least one day a week
your schedule when you do no revision at all. This allows your brain to actively proce
information and move material from short- to long-term memory

Listening to music while you revise can relieve stress. Choose something soothing a
calm to put you in the right frame of mind. If you are becoming very distressed or anxic
let your tutor know immediately and seek support from student services at your univers

The day before the exam, relax and try to enjoy yourself. This will be easier if you ha
organized your revision well and covered all your topics. Finish your revision by lunchti
and organize what you need for the next day. Relax for the remainder of the day, en
a good meal in the evening, have a bath or shower and go to bed early! Make sure y
have some fruit or yoghurt, or fruit and nut mixtures in the house in case you cannot f
breakfast. Allow plenty of time for your journey so that you arrive stress free and ready
perform to the best of your ability.

Take a small lucky mascot into the exam. In times of great stress or mental block, lift y
eyes from your exam paper and focus on the mascot, observe the detail, then look
across the distance of the room, focus on a far wall or out of a window, observe the det
Return your attention to the mascot once more, and then return your attention to
question paper. This simple exercise will give your brain other stimuli to process, wh
may just give the brain the boost it needs to complete your train of thought or get o

that mental block. If you feel the panic rising in the exam, take a long deep breath through your nose and then slowly blow the air out gently through your mouth. Rest your hands, palms facing upwards in your lap until you feel all the tension in your body evaporating.

Tips

- Plan your revision using a schedule, ensuring that you manage your time effectively
- Try to find out as much as you can about the exam beforehand
- Check the university's regulations regarding exams
- Plan to arrive at the exam hall early
- Read the exam questions thoroughly before you answer
- Tackle the questions you know best first
- Think of an emergency plan if you feel you are running out of time
- When the exam is over, resist the temptation to discuss it with your colleagues.

Chapter 19

How to Get the Best Out of the Students' Union

by Elizabeth Huntbach, Mathew Pledger and Maja Dawson

This chapter considers:

- **What a students' union is**
- **The ways in which you can get involved in the students' union**
- **What support the students' union can give you if things do not go as planned**
- **How the students' union can help with academic related problems**
- **The role of student representatives**
- **How the students' union democracy works.**

Introduction

This chapter will focus on the role and the function of a students' union and how studer interact and govern its services. We will explore the individual and collective represe tational services that a students' union provides to its members, focusing specifically the needs of the student community and the regulatory frameworks that govern all giv advice. We will introduce the role of a students' union as an integral component in th process of developing the regulatory frameworks in which the university operates.

To substantiate the chapter we will provide information that will enable you to understar students' union representation and will broadly reflect on the advice, support, and guidan that students' unions' provide.

As a summary we will aim to guide you on how you can access support if your circumstanc change or aspects of your programme do not go as planned.

What a Students' Union Is

When you enrol on to your programme at university, you will automatically become member of the students' union. Students' unions are unique in that they are owned their members – you the student – and you, and your fellow students, will own all of th democratic decisions that are made in the running of the students' union, and the issu that it will campaign for and voice the views of students on.

During your enrolment and induction period at your university you may receive presentation from the students' union. They will outline the services within your studen union, and the opportunities for you to get involved in its activities. If this is not the cas however, you can access your students' union and enquire about its services and activitie

Students' unions will vary in the services that they can provide. You may find that son have a very strong commercial activity, that is, a thriving bar, cafeteria, shops, nightclul and possibly more. Other students' unions may be of a smaller scale, and often primari focus on the ways in which they can effectively represent students.

All services within the students' union will be specifically catered to meet your needs a student. These services may include a reception, a student job centre, bar, activities volunteering centre, an advice centre, a sports centre, or more. Your students' union shou be able to inform you of the services that they have to offer. All you have to commit to doing is visit. If, however, you do find it hard to access the students' union because you are on placement or on another campus, or simply having lots of programme commitments that place demands on your time, your students' union may have a website that can inform you of all its services.

The Ways You Can Get Involved in the Students' Union

There will be a number of ways in which you can get involved in the activities of the students' union. These could be by involving yourself within the democratic side of the students' union by attending the meetings, becoming a student representative, joining a sports club, a special interest, cultural or political society, or even getting involved in the many social activities that are organized for students. You may find, as many students do, that getting involved is a great way to meet fellow like-minded students with similar interests to yourself.

What Support the Students' Union Can Give You

You may find that from time to time there may be issues within your personal life that infringe on your ability to focus on your studies or attend the requirements of your nursing programme, for example lectures, seminars, practice placements. At no point should you ignore these, or keep these problems to yourself. You must tell someone as quickly as possible, so that the university can help you. You may be able to access a students' union adviser who can assist you in ensuring that you tell the right people and follow all the correct procedures to make sure the right decisions are made for you in light of your personal problems.

Students' union advice and assistance is usually given by professionally trained staff that are able to advise on a wide range of issues including providing specialist advice on finance, housing, international student issues, and academic representation issues. If you find that these individuals cannot assist in your case they may provide information on services via access to a wider network of other support services on and off your student campus including careers, counselling, solicitors, study skills, disability issues and so on to which referrals can be made.

The advisers provide an essential service to you that will remain independent from t
university – free, confidential and impartial. To access an adviser you must contact t
students' union. An adviser will have the knowledge of the options that are available t
you when a particular situation arises. An adviser will not tell you what to do, but will a
to empower you to help you take ownership of your problem, and help you decide a w
to obtain a suitable resolution.

On making contact with a students' union adviser most will start to compile a file of yo
case in order that there are contact details for you and a history of key documents, su
as letters from the university, and a record of the meetings. The adviser will usually wc
within the framework in which you have given him or her permission to represent yc
This will normally be carried out through your signing a declaration that the adviser
representing you and that you are authorizing him or her to discuss your case with membe
of university staff and other organizations should there need to be any clarification
issues. However, it should be noted that by your signing a declaration, and by givi
permission for an adviser of the students' union to represent you, that this does not me
that you can relinquish your responsibilities. The adviser will discuss with university st
and occasionally attend meetings on your behalf if you are unable to make the meeti
for a good reason. However, it is still your responsibility to keep up to date with what
happening with your case.

The information that is held on your file is confidential and usually a students' uni
will have a confidentiality policy as to whom the adviser can discuss your case wi
Confidentiality policies usually enable the adviser to discuss your case in confidence wi
another students' union adviser or manager of the service in order that any areas whe
the adviser may need further support or confirmation are covered. Information held
the adviser is subject to the law of the land and you are entitled to request copies of th
information under the Data Protection Act. In many cases confidentiality is only extende
usually with your permission, if it is believed that you are a danger to yourself or others.

You will find that most advisers will represent students in a number of ways. The ide
way to discuss your case would be within a face-to-face interview setting; however, mc
advisers will be prepared to offer advice and guidance via the telephone or e-mail. Plea
note that any method of communicating with an adviser other than a face-to-face intervie
could affect case confidentiality and the quality of support that is offered to you.

Most advisers will provide a representation service on an appointment system to ensu
that students are given adequate time to deal with their problem. You may find, howev

that your students' union holds a 'drop-in' facility for you to quickly access an adviser prior to making an appointment. To find out if this service is available to you, you must contact your students' union, or access the students' union website.

Although advisers are usually able to give advice in a number of different ways, to ensure that you can access an adviser and have the opportunity of obtaining students' union representation you should access the service early. Do not leave your case to the last minute as an adviser may not be able to represent you.

How the Students' Union Can Help With Academic Related Problems

Once you enrol on your programme you will automatically be responsible and obliged to follow a set of university regulations. These regulations govern all of the activities of the university and will inform you of your rights as a student. You must ensure that you familiarize yourself with these regulations and conform to them at all times during your programme. The students' union will assist you in any queries that you may have within these regulations.

While on your programme, you may at some point experience some academic difficulties which may lead you to being subjected to university procedures as outlined within your regulations, for example you may be asked to attend a disciplinary hearing over an alleged breach of the university regulations, such as allegations of plagiarism.

The representation that a students' union adviser will provide to you in this instance would include representation within university meetings/hearings and advice, support and guidance in preparing your case. Within the hearing the adviser will ensure that the university regulations are followed and that you have the opportunity of a fair hearing. On a different level the adviser will also be there as emotional support at a time when you may feel particularly anxious.

Alongside your university's regulations, the Nursing and Midwifery Council (NMC) has set standards of nursing care, which are found within a Code of Professional Conduct (NMC 2002; NMC 2004). As a student nurse you will not only be responsible for following the university regulations, but you will also be expected to practise and follow the NMC Code of Professional Conduct. You will not be a registered nurse so will not be held to account by the NMC, but be expected to act within the spirit of these at all times. If you do breach one

of these standards the university may take this very seriously, and investigate the mat
through their own internal procedures.

Academic appeals

There are nationally set codes of practice on how universities should facilitate academ
appeals. Most universities will have, as part of their procedures, mechanisms for you
make an appeal and have a hearing to an independent senior panel within the univers
There are two grounds of appeal within most universities. Firstly, on the basis that the
was a material irregularity in how you were assessed. For example, if there were changes
the published guidelines for a particular assessment about which you were not inform
The second, and most common, ground for appeal is that there were special circumstan
that the assessment board did not know about that affected your performance in th
assessment, such as illness, homelessness or any other serious circumstances that cou
not have been foreseen.

No university will allow you to appeal an assessment result on the basis that you disag
with the decision of the assessor. This would be an appeal against the academic judgeme
of the university. This is because your university will have clear methods and procedu
in place for ensuring that the assessment policies on your programme are fair, transpare
and robust. For example, your university will have been audited by external professio
organizations, including the NMC, which will have resulted in their giving appro
regarding the quality of your programme. Furthermore, your university will have exter
examiners who are drawn from other universities and professional organizations that
there to ensure commonality of standards across the country. Please note that while th
have been cases in which students have challenged academic judgements in court,
student to date has been successful in legally challenging an academic decision.

Complaints

You may experience issues while studying on your programme, and wish to lodg
complaint in an attempt to resolve your concerns. Complaints will normally entail a let
of complaint being submitted to a senior named individual within the university. T
letter normally will have to outline your current student details, the rationale behind
complaint, the complaint itself, the steps that you have taken in order to try and reso
the issue(s), and your desired way in which the complaint should be resolved.

Once you have submitted your complaint, the complaint may then be facilitated by
named individual, who may conduct an investigation that will look into the nature of y

complaint. The named individual should not be involved in your teaching or support, so will remain impartial throughout. Following the investigation you will receive a written response notifying you of the outcome of your complaint. If you have exhausted all your university complaints procedures, you may wish to pursue your complaint to the Office of Independent Adjudicator (OIA). Your students' union should be able to offer guidance on this.

One key thing to remember is that the advisers that assist you in your case will be independent, impartial, and non-judgemental. Do not feel anxious in approaching these people. They are there to help, support and guide you. If they cannot help you through your problem, they will have the knowledge to signpost you to an appropriate service which can help.

The Role of Student Representatives

Your university will have a number of methods for gathering feedback from you and your cohort of students. Your views of your experience on the programme and the quality of your programme are important in order that your university is responsive to the needs of students. Many universities have a student representative system whereby a number of student representatives are elected to represent different intakes and branches of the programme. These representatives meet on a regular basis with the members of university staff who run and support the programme. It is important that your views are sought in all areas of programme planning, content and delivery. Student representatives sometimes find that issues that they raise regarding their programme of study do not always effect change during their time on the programme; however, they may affect later intakes. The student voice on programme committees is critical and can often effect significant change to areas such as timetabling, placements and hand-in dates to name a few examples.

How the Students' Union Democracy Works

The students' union is a democratic membership organization. All activities and areas of the students' union operations are accountable to the student community. The democratic structures of the union can often be quite complex, yet will feed into the key decision making committees of the students' union, union council/union senate.

There will be one committee meeting of the students' union that will be responsible for policy creation and approval. The committee's main function is to ensure accountability

for the elected officers, set union policy, and mandate the elected officers to focus th
energy on particular projects, for example campaigns.

In most cases, any student can attend these committees. To find out when and where th
are held, you can contact your students' union. By attending, this will be an opportunity
you to input and voice how you would like to see your students' union run. You will ha
the opportunity to tell them what issues you feel they should be active in campaigning c

Your students' union will be run by a group of elected officers. These officers will be elect
by students at your university to campaign on issues that are pertinent and represe
the views of students. The amount and the roles of these officers will differ betwe
universities. There will often be a number of full-time elected officers and part-time elect
officers that are elected for a set period of time, usually a year, to lead the students' uni

To assist the elected officers, most students' unions are affiliated to the National Union
Students (NUS). This is an organization that represents the views and national intere
of students studying within the United Kingdom. There are a number of benefits to yc
students' union being affiliated to NUS, one of the obvious ones is the opportunity for
students to obtain an NUS card entitling the owner to various discounts within a numl
of high street shops and outlets.

The students' union is independent from the university and has the opportunity
directly affect the decisions that are made within the university. The students' union is
organization that represents the student community and will therefore play an integ
role when the university is reviewing its rules and regulations on the conduct of studer
The feedback that the students' union provides is specifically student focused and will a
to ensure that the processes that the university put in place are fair and transparent a
there is equality of treatment for all students across the university.

The elected officers are responsible for strengthening links with the university a
will provide representation of the student community through sitting on a range
committees, working groups or steering groups to ensure that the university takes i
account the student perspective. This generally means that your views are expres
at senior committees of your university by the elected representatives of your studer
union. Any decision made by the university that may affect your student experience
be consulted on with the students' union which will endeavour to ensure that it takes i
account your needs as a student.

TIPS

- Find out about the work and facilities available at your students' union
- Investigate where on the campus your students' union is located
- Think about how you might be actively involved in the union
- If you need representation, contact an adviser as soon as possible.

References

NMC (2002) *An NMC Guide for Students of Nursing and Midwifery.* London, NMC. Available at: www.nmc-uk.org/aFrameDisplay.aspx?DocumentID=1896

NMC (2004) *The NMC Code of Professional Conduct: Standards for Conduct, Performance and Ethics.* London, NMC. Available at: www.nmc-uk.org/aFrameDisplay .aspx?DocumentID=201

Chapter 20

Getting Support from Your Personal Tutor

by Steve Trenoweth and Helen Robson

This chapter considers:

- **How to get to know your personal tutor**
- **How you might contact your personal tutor**
- **What support your tutor can offer you**
- **How to manage your time effectively with your tutor.**

Introduction

Of all the people that you will meet on your programme and all the people that you work with, your personal tutor can be a pivotal figure in helping you to be successful. or she can also be important in aiding your development as a competent and professic healthcare practitioner. It is worth spending some time thinking about what you mi need from your personal tutor and how you might go about developing a product working relationship with him or her.

Getting to Know Your Personal Tutor

At the start of your programme you will be assigned a personal tutor, and it is lik that they will want to meet up with you for an introductory interview. This will of involve discussing with you any concerns you might have or to clarify issues relating to programme. They will almost certainly want to discuss with you the role they will undert to support you in your studies and it is a good idea to discuss not only what you expec them but what they also expect of you. You might agree a 'learning contract', which s out a clear plan about what you personally would like to achieve on the programme, a when you will meet up with your tutor.

When you meet up with your tutor during your programme, it is very helpful to give th an update on your progress and what some of the issues have been for you since you s them last. Try not to assume that they know everything that has been happening to y We often are approached by our personal students who start by saying 'You remem two years ago when I was off sick with the flu. . . '. In reality, the answer might well be Your tutor will have responsibilities to many students, and while each student is, of cou very important, it is not always possible to remember every detail of every one – so d be offended if they look at you blankly!

Contacting Your Personal Tutor

This might seem a minor point but it is important to find out how you might contact y personal tutor.

Some tutors might well offer an open-door policy and welcome you at any time or t may 'ring fence' certain times during the day or week to see their personal students. So and this is much more likely, would prefer that you made an appointment to see them. As much as tutors would like to offer a 'drop-in' facility, this is often not possible given their workload. It is important to bear in mind that your tutor's responsibilities are many and varied. They will almost certainly have responsibilities to other groups of students, often not only to pre-registration learners, but to post-registration learners as well. They might be undertaking research. They will inevitably have a variety of teaching commitments and will have to attend meetings that compete for their time.

So, it is a good idea to check with your personal tutor how they would like to be contacted by you. If they would like you to make an appointment to see them, should you contact them via e-mail, phone or write to them? We imagine that most tutors, like us, would prefer to be e-mailed.

However, if you have an unforeseen emergency, then your personal tutor will try their best to see you as soon as they possibly can.

What Support Does Your Tutor Offer?

Each university has a slightly different model so it is best to find out exactly what support your personal tutor is able to offer. However, in broad terms your tutor can offer the following.

Pastoral support

Healthcare programmes can be personally and professionally challenging. They can be demanding and intense. You might, for example, encounter people and situations that remind you of difficult times in your own life and bring back painful memories. You might have been moved or disturbed by some of the situations you encounter while on clinical placement. Alternatively, you might have failed some aspect of your programme and have had your confidence knocked as a result.

Whatever the reason there might be times during your programme when you need a sympathetic ear and need some emotional support. It is very important that you are able to discuss problems and issues if and as they arise. Don't let things build up!

While the role of personal tutor is not that of a counsellor, they can and will listen. They are healthcare professionals and will understand. It is important to remember that they

have also undertaken healthcare education and indeed may have had similar issues to y
during their own training.

If they are unable to offer you the help that they feel you need, they might recomme
that you see, in complete confidence, a counsellor or other service within the univers
that may be able to help.

Academic support

Many students who commence healthcare programmes may not have studied a
university before. For some, their only experience of education may be when they were
school.

To study at a university, for some, might understandably seem a daunting prospect! Inde
the language used sometimes can seem strange – you are asked to reflect, critically analy
evaluate and so on. You might feel it necessary to have a chat to someone who will
able to help you navigate your way through the academic component of the programn
In the first instance, you might like to discuss this with your personal tutor if you feel y
are in need of academic support and guidance.

Please remember, though, that the time available for your personal tutor may be limit
and they may not be able to spend as much time helping you to develop academica
as they would like. They will, however, be able to recommend services, such as learni
skills support centres or other resources if they feel you need extra academic support. Th
might also ask you to have a chat with the university's disability team.

If your tutor is able to offer academic support, and is happy to discuss a particular theoreti
assignment with you, it is best to think of this as having an academic dialogue or a cl
about the issue rather than asking them what you need to do in order to pass! That
don't expect your tutor to give you the answers but use your tutor to bounce ideas off. Y
may, of course, ask their advice if you feel you might not have the correct focus. Your tu
might suggest or direct you to a particular piece of research or literature and we wou
strongly advise you to seek this out.

One last thing, unless your tutor has asked you to do this, do not e-mail or leave an es:
on their desk expecting them to read it for you before you submit it!

Practical advice

There are many policies and procedures relating to your programme, and your university has many opportunities available to you that you may not be aware of. Of course, you will be unable to access services that can support you if you are unaware of them. For example, you might have been diagnosed with a particular disability, such as dyslexia, and need information about how you can obtain the learning support you require. Your personal tutor will be able to point you in the right direction.

Please remember that your tutor can only help you if you bring to their attention problems and issues that you are having and which might affect your programme. One area in particular your tutor will need to be aware of is major changes to your health status which will affect your studies, particularly if you have been recently diagnosed with a health problem or become pregnant.

You might be having particular difficulties relating to the programme or in your life in general. Your personal tutor can clarify and explore with you the various options available. For example, if you are having genuine difficulties, it might be that you require additional time to submit your theoretical assignments. It might be that your tutor suggests that you take a short break from the programme so that you can concentrate on problems at home. Your tutor will be able to discuss with you the relevant policies and procedures and guide you through the process.

Before seeing your personal tutor, however, it is worth your while to look through your handbooks and other literature you will have been given at the start of your programme. It is likely that most of the information you are looking for can be found there. However, if you require confirmation or clarification about any of the issues then make an appointment to see your tutor.

Support if it all goes wrong

Sometimes, and fortunately rarely, a student's behaviour or conduct may give rise to a complaint. As healthcare professionals, we must be able to justify our actions and the decisions that we take. It might be that accusations of plagiarism have been levelled against you or a complaint may arise from your conduct while on a clinical placement. Your tutor will be able to advise you whom to contact for support, and how to contact them if you are unsure. At the very least, they will advise you to contact your students' union. However, be aware that your tutor is unable to represent you at investigatory or disciplinary hearin and will be unable to comment on the specific allegations made against you.

Monitoring your progress

During your programme, your personal tutor may ask to see you or you may have decid at the start of your programme to meet up at certain points in order to discuss yc progress. Often these are at 'milestone' points on the programme to see how you getting along. These are important opportunities for your personal reflection and grow as a healthcare practitioner.

At such times, your tutor will discuss your achievements and successes as well as thir that have not gone so well for you. It is important for you to able to be honest with yourse but you should not be afraid to talk about what you see as your strengths and share sor of the good things that have happened to you on the programme.

The important thing is that in monitoring your progress you and your tutor will ne to have an honest and critical appraisal and you should see this in professional terr Please remember that if your tutor is being critical, or challenges you on a particular poi that this is directed towards your personal and professional development as a healthca practitioner. For example, it might be that they feel you are not working to your potential and they need you to reflect on this. By all means, state your case if you do agree, but remember your tutor is merely trying to help you.

Also, remember that as much as we would all like to be told only the good things abc ourselves, we require a balanced view of both our developmental needs and our streng in order to progress and grow as practitioners.

We would also suggest that when you meet up with your personal tutor to moni your progress, that you write up the outcomes and include this in a portfolio or take t opportunity to review your personal development plan.

At the end of the programme your personal tutor may also be able to offer advice for pc registration education and development opportunities, or indeed, to help you identify a plan a career pathway. At the end of your programme, it is expected that your Perso Tutor will respond to requests for an academic reference.

Managing Your Time Effectively with Your Personal Tutor

It is unlikely that you will have unlimited time with your personal tutor and it is most likely you will have a limited period of time to discuss issues. It is important, therefore, for you to be able to manage your time with your tutor effectively. There are a few things we would like to suggest here. Firstly, be aware of the time frame and be businesslike. Next, be active and not passive. Here, you may like to come with an agenda or a list of items that you wish to discuss.

If you have come for academic support, perhaps as you would like help with a particular assessment, then make sure you at least come with some ideas or a plan. If you could come with something concrete like a 'spider diagram' this would help your tutor to understand where you are coming from.

Tips

- Think of your tutor as an adviser and a guide rather than as someone who will solve your problems
- Try to make an appointment with your tutor rather than dropping in (unless your tutor is happy with this)
- Don't let things build up! Make time to see your tutor at the first sign of trouble
- Be mindful of the many and varied duties your tutor has
- Be time aware and plan your time with your tutor effectively
- Take on board any feedback offered and see this in professional terms.

Section 5

Preparing for Your Nursing/Midwifery Career

In this final section, the authors help you to consider your own personal and professional change and development, both within the programme and beyond.

Change is an essential part of succeeding in nursing and midwifery education. Undoubtedly you will develop new knowledge and skills. You may also find that some of your views and beliefs have changed. This section helps you to consider how the change process might affect you. In so doing, you will be paving the way for the final change process in your programme – that of qualifying and commencing your nursing or midwifery career. In Chapter 22 the author will help you to consider how you might best prepare yourself for this transition from student nurse or midwife to qualified healthcare practitioner, and how you might secure your ideal post. Chapter 23 bids you to pursue excellence and lifelong learning in your career.

Chapter 21

Personal Change

by David Stroud and Steve Trenoweth

In this chapter you will:

- **Develop an understanding of the implications of your own personal change**
- **Consider the possible impact that working in healthcare environments can have on the concept of self**
- **Consider the positive and negative effects of personal change**
- **Learn how to manage the change process.**

Introduction

During your nursing/midwifery education, you will develop important skills not only your clinical practice but also essential life skills. Indeed, it is not unusual for students nursing and midwifery to comment that they feel they have changed on a personal level process which is not always easy or straightforward. So, independent of the aims of y programme you might gradually realize that you are becoming more self-confident, will to take calculated risks in personal relationships, and able to assert yourself by stating wh you want, by saying no, by expressing your own opinion and so on. This can be quit subtle process and often the first hint of this might come from others commenting abc the change in you.

Besides helping you develop skills and knowledge, nursing/midwifery education aims challenge your attitudes and the way you perceive relevant issues such as health, illn and human relationships. Mezirow (1977) calls this 'perspective transformation', and it affect your personal as well as your professional life.

In this chapter, we help you to capitalize on positive changes that are likely to occur wh meeting some of the challenges that might result from the change process.

The Change Process

If you have ever tried to get rid of an unwanted habit you know how easy it is for it to retur you let your guard down too soon. It's the same with personal change – there is a tende to go back to former ways of thinking, feeling and acting. Kurt Lewin is one of the m influential writers on change, and his theory of unfreeze–move–refreeze is applica to the aims of nursing/midwifery programmes. Put simply, unfreeze means becom aware of the present situation and the need for change; moving means implementing changes; and refreezing means consolidating the changes and making them perman (Lewin 1947).

To achieve these aims, there will be an emphasis on self-awareness throughout programme, which includes an awareness of how you are changing. Your program requires you to monitor this change in reflective accounts in your personal developm plan and in supervision. Other places where you're required to demonstrate and record s awareness is in your theoretical assignments and clinical placement books. Furtherm there may be feedback in class from your lecturer and fellow students when you do presentations, and from your clinical placement mentors and reflective supervisors. Try not to be defensive or dismiss comments and feedback as these can be an important way in which you develop that all important self-insight. Indeed, other people are often vital to our understanding of how we are changing and, as the psychiatrist Harry Stack Sullivan (1953) suggested, it is not possible to develop awareness in isolation.

Personal Change in Nursing

There have been many studies (such as Benner 1984, Melia 1987 and Ferguson and Hope 1999) which have catalogued how student nurses and midwives develop during their pre-registration education. What is abundantly clear is that personal change is a central feature of this process – that is, it is most likely that you will change. Certainly, you will learn new skills and develop a specialist body of knowledge that will be essential for your professional clinical practice. You may also change some of your ideas and beliefs about health and illness or, indeed, life in general.

Some of the experiences you will have during your nursing/midwifery education will be poignant or remarkable, and will no doubt leave a lasting impression. When we recall our own training, we still think of some of the people that we tried to care for. We also remember our feelings of being unable to help as much as we would like owing to our lack of experience at that time, and how inadequate that made us feel. Feelings like this cannot but have an impact on us as people. But these experiences are inevitable and important – they help us to develop and grow as people. They spur us on to know more and to develop our skills, so that if such situations were to occur again, we are prepared.

Change, then, is an essential and necessary part of your education. However, it may not always be clear to you that you are changing – but to those around you, it may be all too obvious. Undoubtedly, the personal change you experience will be positive but it is important to be mindful of your personal and professional development as such awareness allows you to take steps to offset any potential challenging consequences of this process.

Positive Effects of Change

Without question, your clinical experiences are the most important factor which helps you to develop your identity as a nurse or midwife and it is here where your profession

takes on its most profound meaning for you. Your interactions with role models, peers a
patients/clients are crucial in the development of your professional identity.

To start off with, it is likely you will want to learn the 'rules' of nursing/midwifery, tha
the very basic and fundamental skills and knowledge which you require within your o
speciality, such as how to give an injection; how to take a pulse; how to respond to a cli
who is experiencing auditory hallucinations and so forth. That is, you will develop
knowledge and skills in your own speciality in order to be able to make a real difference
someone's life. Helping someone to improve their life, and indeed, being able to help sa
someone's life, comprises a remarkable set of skills, the acquisition of which you sho
celebrate. As a result you will hopefully grow in self-confidence to deliver care to the
who require your help.

Research seems to indicate that those who facilitate your learning, such as your lectur
and mentors, will at first also encourage you to develop your knowledge and understand
of rules. These rules are very important as they can contain essential information that
help you to develop the art of caring. Some rules cannot be found in books and are of
essential to the smooth delivery of care – the useful tips, rules of thumb which experien
nurses have developed from their own practice and experience.

Over time, it is likely that you will be so familiar with these rules that they will become
everyday part of your life! You may not even be aware of them. You will be able to perfc
tasks in a matter-of-fact way that is likely to leave your students astonished. Skilled, exp
nurses and midwives have the ability to perform complex tasks seemingly effortlessly – a
they seem to be perceptive and astute when it comes to their clinical assessments a
empathic in their understanding of their clients' needs.

Increasingly, nurses and midwives are being encouraged to utilize evidence in their clin
practice, as well as being able to capitalize on the richness and value of knowledge whic
embedded in their own personal experience. You might witness an extraordinarily ski
intervention by a qualified nurse or midwife, and when you ask them to explain what t
did they might dismiss this as common sense. That is, they seem to be oblivious to
depth and quality of their skills, and the range of their knowledge which has allowed th
to respond effectively and expertly to a complex clinical situation.

It is a shame, however, that some gifted clinical nurses and midwives (and indeed stude
are not aware of their own personal change and their own personal journey to expert
and that they dismiss their talents as something anyone could do! Such nurses

midwives, it has been suggested, require (and deserve) support to be able to reflect upon and develop personal awareness of their professional development and growth. But consider this – in a few years' time, you will have the same question posed by one of your own students, and you may also be tempted to say 'it is common sense'. However, don't fall into the trap which so many other talented nurses/midwives have done over the years – reflect upon your change. Take some time out and consider how far you have travelled!

It is essential that you are supported in your attempts to make sense of your experiences and to put them into perspective so that you are able to learn from them. It is also important that you are able to articulate and explore your feelings, particularly when you encounter clinical events which seem out of keeping with your expectations. Sometimes, the theory may seem out of place with the practice. And, of course, the practice may seem out of place with the theory. You may feel torn between the two here and there is some suggestion from research that students learn to conform to the rules, and to use different types of knowledge, in the university and in clinical practice. This is obviously not an ideal situation. It is through psychological support, reflection and discussion with others, such as your mentor, clinical staff and tutors, that it is possible to discuss and resolve tensions that can arise.

An essential skill for nurses/midwives in order to fully and effectively respond to a client's needs (and to make a full contribution to multiprofessional working) is being assertive. Here, it may be necessary to challenge decisions made by other members of the clinical team if you feel they are not in the client's best interest. Students undergoing positive change often report that they feel more assertive – able to say no, to truthfully express their needs, wants, likes and dislikes, and to be more honest with people in general.

You might also find that the analytical skills you develop in clinical situations, and your understanding of people (their wants and needs), become useful, or transferable, to your life in general. You might find yourself wanting to see beyond the obvious to try to understand the underlying issues in events that affect you in your personal life, or even world events. Simple solutions or simple answers to complex problems in the world might seem a bit too convenient! You might find yourself trying to understand what really lies behind a news headline, or why a friend might have become angry with you and so forth. You might well become more aware of and sympathetic to human suffering. That is, in a whole range of issues, both clinically and personally, you might find that your perspective has been transformed!

In short, you might well find yourself, as a result of the nursing/midwifery educatic becoming more self-reliant and independent in your thinking. You might feel more able meet life's challenges. You might find yourself being more able to compromise with peopl being more receptive to their perspective and views. Having a more analytical approac to life can help you make better informed choices not only in the clinical environment b also in your life in general. Furthermore, you will certainly develop transferable skills, su as developing writing, numeracy and verbal skills, using information technology, tea working and so forth. Such changes can have a profound and positive effect on our ov self-esteem and self-worth as individuals.

Negative Effects of Change

When you first start in your nursing/midwifery career (and possible when you start to wo in clinical services) you might well experience anticipatory anxiety – fear of the unknow You will understandably want to create a good impression for fear of being judge negatively by staff. There will be pressure upon you to fit in – to adjust to the rhythms ar flow of clinical environments or clinical situations, that is, to conform to the rules of th culture, organization or profession. We are social animals and most of us have a desire belong, and it is understandable that we would want to conform to the rules of our chose profession. This is a natural process and often occurs when we are faced with situatior in which we feel out of place. Sometimes, you may feel you have learnt more about th routines of a particular clinical service, than actual care.

To some extent we all need to acclimatize to the clinical environment or service that we a joining. However, there are dangers of blindly conforming, that is, of unthinkingly trying fit into an occupational or organizational culture. Being compliant with others' wishes h implications for your own personal change and indeed professional practice. Furthermor we are in danger of copying and picking up colleagues' bad habits or slavishly following th rules. Modern nursing and midwifery isn't about conformity – in fact, it is about challengir existing ways of working! In a modern healthcare system, we are required to question o understanding of health and illness, so that we are able to grow as professionals and, mo importantly, we are able to provide care which is based on sound methods and actir in our clients' best interests – not what is most convenient for us. So, when you 'go wit the flow', your focus is on *not* personally changing. In fact, it is about doing what othe want you to do rather than what you feel, as a professional, is the right thing to do. This not always an easy thing to do – but if you want to develop as a practitioner, to provic effective, modern care, it is essential!

You will inevitably encounter people who will die; who are living with profound disabilities; who are trying to cope with illnesses and disease. We cannot, and should not, fail to be moved. It is likely that we will consider how we might live with such problems – we might even become painfully aware of how transient and how fragile life actually is. We might start our own quest for the meaning of our lives, and perhaps even life in general. When we started out on our nursing careers we recall distinctly being aware of this. However, this helped and encouraged us to see the world in a new way and enabled us to put our own lives into perspective. Yes, life can be temporary and painful, but our life is for living – so let's try to make the best of it. 'Carpe diem', wrote the Roman poet Horace – seize the day.

Change can sometimes be a painful process. It is natural and understandable that we should, in seeking to protect ourselves, try to resist personal change.

Strange as it may sound, people resist change even when it is for the better. It's a case of 'better the devil you know than the one you don't'. Hans Seyle (1946), the father of stress research, came to the conclusion that any change, positive or negative, had to be adapted to, and can therefore cause stress. So not only is a brush with the law stressful, but so is the wedding of your dreams!

Resisting our own change can cause additional problems for us. For example, if change is needed we might try to control and change those around us, that is, try to force others to change to be more like us so that we don't have to change! However, it is unlikely that people will willingly do our bidding, or conform to our perspective, and they might well resist our attempts to change them. Such people might well often find themselves in conflict with others. Without an awareness of how our ideas about ourselves and our lives might be changing, we might unfairly project our anxiety or anger on to other people.

This has implications for our own personal boundaries. Without support we might be tempted to protect ourselves, psychologically. We might 'build a psychological wall' through which no painful experiences can penetrate. That is, we might try to distance ourselves emotionally from others. While this might protect us, we might seem to others to be uncaring and unfeeling. Certainly, this has a grave implication for the care process. If we are emotionally distant then we are likely to lack the capacity for understanding and empathy – key features of any clinical input in nursing and midwifery.

It is important to have boundaries between your private life and your life as a student. For instance, you must maintain patient confidentiality, including with your family and close friends. But remember there is bound to be some permeation between your two worlds.

Adverse events in your personal life might negatively affect you at university or on clinic placement, and vice versa. Yet one world can benefit from the other – what happens your personal life can help you cope with problems in the clinical area or understar complex ideas in lectures, and the converse is also true.

A very important issue is that you might be changing but those around you do ne Students sometimes say that those closest to them have noticed changes – and this ca be an extremely positive thing. It can also be negative if not handled well. To yo friends, families and partners you may seem a 'different' person. Sometimes, people fir themselves questioning their current lifestyle and as a consequence they may feel th their priorities in life have changed.

It is advisable to listen to, and even solicit, impressions of how you are changing fro those close to you. You may be surprised by what you hear! However, if you ask them f feedback, make it clear that you want it to be truthful. Listen to what they have to say ar try to empathize with their perspective. It is through understanding the needs of tho significant to us that we can undertake the necessary steps to ensure that our persor and professional changes are positive.

Final Thoughts

The key to managing your personal change then is to be aware of how you are changing. O advice is not to avoid or ignore these changes. Manage them, and the concomitant stre proactively. Furthermore, an important way of changing is being able to respond effective to personal and professional challenges, which can arise from the nursing/midwife education, and being able to put experiences into perspective.

Tips

- Be proactive! Be aware of how you might be changing
- Understand and appreciate the importance of change
- Understand the impact of your change on others close to you
- Talk to your family and friends
- Get support from your personal tutor or mentor.

References

Benner, P. (1984) *From Novice to Expert: Excellence and Power in Clinical Nursing Practice.* Menlo Park, Addison-Wesley.

Ferguson, K. and Hope, K. (1999) From novice to competent practitioner: tracking the progress of undergraduate mental health nurses. *Journal of Advanced Nursing,* **29**(3), 630–8.

Lewin, K. (1947) Frontiers in group dynamics. *Human Relations,* **1**, 5–42.

Melia, K. (1987) *Learning and Working: The Occupational Socialisation of Nurses.* London, Tavistock Publications.

Mezirow, J. (1977) Perspective transformation. *Studies in Adult Education,* **9**(2), 153–7.

Seyle H. (1946) The general adaptation syndrome and the diseases of adaptation. *J Clin Endocrinol. Metab.,* **6**, 117–230.

Sullivan, H.S. (1953) <u>*The Interpersonal Theory Of Psychiatry*</u>. New York, Norton.

Chapter 22

Preparing Yourself for Your Nursing/Midwifery Career

by Samantha Torres

This chapter considers:

- **What the right post for you is**
- **How to apply for the post and prepare for the interview**
- **How to support yourself in the transition from student to nurse/midwife**
- **How to maintain your portfolio and develop your career.**

Introduction

You have just spent three years in nursing or midwifery education and during that t
you may have wished it was all over quickly! But now it is over and being a student d
not seem that bad after all. The reality has set in and now you are a professional – so
accountable for your practice. To start off with this can be a daunting and unnerv
experience. I know how that might feel as I have been there – and not too long
either! Therefore, it is vital that you support yourself from the start and continue to
so throughout your career. If you assert yourself and utilize all the resources and supp
networks available to you, you will be a successful high flying professional with an ongc
passion for nursing or midwifery!

The Right Post

I bet the first thing that comes to your mind is money! However, while money motivate
in our posts there are several other factors that you may or may not have considered. Y
first post as a novice staff nurse or midwife is a vital and important stepping stone in y
career. It is the foundation to what makes you a professional and shapes your practice.

You might be looking for a post with an employer that you have been in touch with
a student by having clinical placements there. Your experience in that time has been
influential factor, which is great, but you need to think about your role now and how
will change when you join them in the workforce. What was it about the experience? W
how the team worked and supported each other or did you find management suppor
and accommodating for example? Was that because you were a student and they w
flexible? Maybe staff working there did not feel the same as you.

You might be familiar with your potential employer or not it but it is worth checking
their commitment to employees via their websites or human resources department. If
already have a specific department in mind why not give them a call and ask to be sho
around.

You have to think about the location of the service and how long it is going to take
to get there. You cannot afford to be tired before getting to work as eventually y
performance will be affected. It could be that your route to work seems to have more t
its fair share of road works. Your shift pattern will also play a part. Is it 9 a.m.–5 p.m., e

or late shifts? Are you expected to work rotational shifts (i.e. from day to night duty)? If so, what impact might this have on you and your family?

It could be that travelling and location of shift patterns are not factors but your home life is just as it was when you were a student. Remember those days of balancing being a parent and arranging child care. You will have to consider this even more when you are employed as it is most unlikely they will be casually accommodating as they were when your were a student by letting you do 9 a.m. – 5 p.m. on your four week placement!

You might want to find out if they have a flexible working policy which will assist travelling or childcare arrangements in the long run. That is fine, but what about the school's summer holidays? Most employers run childcare schemes during the holidays that you pay a reasonable fee for, so your children can have fun and you can go to work without worrying who is going to look after them. But remember: as a staff nurse, your employer expects a commitment from you as they need to think about minimizing disruption to the service – so do investigate these issues carefully beforehand.

In order for you to develop as a professional, you may want to consider the availability of post-registration education and support. Remember that this not only includes courses but programmes such as preceptorship and clinical supervision. You might want to find out what the employer provides as mandatory and statutory training as well as internal and external training opportunities. You might want to ask these questions to the team members and find out if the department is conducive to lifelong learning. Try to find out if there is a waiting list for training and if you are given study leave.

Job Application

So you think you have found the right post and they are looking for staff. Time management is very important now – from receiving the application to completing it and sending it off. You do not want any unnecessary stress.

The key to successful application forms is to use those theoretical skills you learnt in university. Analyse the person specification and job description and ask yourself what they are looking for. This will help you to tell them that you are the right person for the post.

The job description will tell you much about what is expected in the role while the job specification is normally split into essential or desirable criteria that you should have. The trick is to pick up on what they expect, what you have done or can do, and put it across the supporting information section on the application form. Being brief, factual and to point is essential as this will determine if you are short-listed for the post or not. Equa accurate spelling, grammar, punctuation and general neatness of the application form (to get it word processed if you can) will really tell the recruitment and selection pa about you and will show that you have an eye for detail.

You might want to consider looking back on some of your portfolio material during yo nursing and midwifery programme as you most likely completed personal and professio development plans. Use some of those strengths or areas for development you highlight and think if some of them are still valid and worth mentioning. Remember your skills transferable and always need to be developed further. In some cases, a curriculum vit might be requested or appropriate to support your application. Dig out the one you wro while studying, update it and send it off!

Interview Preparation

You have been invited for the interview so you need to get cracking with preparation. Lo back on the job specification and job description and start highlighting the key them and think about the questions you are likely to be asked. To help you ask staff member they remember the types of question they were asked. You might want to enlist a frie so you can do some mock interviews.

You might be asked to bring your portfolio, copies of educational certificates and yo Nursing and Midwifery personal identification number (PIN) so make sure these are all a safe place. Some interviews may request a presentation so make sure you are prepare practise well and have all the materials printed. You might need to find out beforeha the presentation facilities they have available, such as an overhead projector.

This might be the time to ensure that you are fully up to date on developments in yo speciality. Spend some time looking at recent research and policy initiatives that you fe might come up in the interview. If you have not done so already arrange an informal vi to the department or service to get a feel of the place and see how the team works. A yourself if you can see yourself working there before you proceed.

Your interview is a week away and you need to be making sure now exactly where it and how you are going to get there. Do a trial journey if necessary as time is crucial a being late will make you stressed and perform badly in the interview. The day before the interview is a time when you need to relax – that does not mean working an extra bank shift – and get plenty of sleep too. You need to get your smart clothes ready and ironed at least the day before. Remember first impression counts!

It is the day and you have arrived in ample time, well done you! So you are nervous and if you were late you would have been a complete mess.

The interview is about you so it is your opportunity to sell yourself and the key here is honesty throughout. During the interview the panel will expect you to be nervous – this is not uncommon so try not to be embarrassed about this. You might want to say to the panel that you are feeling nervous – you will usually find that they will try to put you at your ease.

When you are answering questions, be clear and to the point and be aware of eye contact and your body posture. You want to show them that you are interested and want to get this post so looking keen and enthusiastic is paramount here. Quite often interviewees do not listen to the questions so pay attention otherwise you will end up talking around the subject and lose marks.

Remember you did all the reading and research in preparation for the interview – well now is the time to mention this! However, remember it is not what you know but what knowledge you can apply to clinical practice. Sounds familiar from university days? Remember, being a professional is about having relevant knowledge and being able to use this to deliver high quality nursing/midwifery care. You should use previous experiences as a student to answer the questions but this is where the honesty comes in. You will not lose marks if you have not had the experience but stating what you would do in that situation is just as important. You might even be asked to explain further something you mentioned in your application form – honesty is definitely the best policy. If you are unable to answer a question, then whatever you do don't bluff! You will be rumbled straight away! Instead, admit this, but say that you will spend some time researching this area to ensure that you are fully up to date.

Going for an interview is about being asked questions but, significantly, at the end you have the opportunity to ask questions too. You should use this opportunity to raise questions on areas that have been discussed in this chapter such as flexible working policies, childcare arrangements, preceptorship programme, their clinical and managerial

supervision structure, further education possibilities and, most importantly, when and h
will you find out if you have been successful.

Getting the Right Support

You are now a staff nurse or midwife literally overnight. You feel out of your depth a
you might even find yourself still saying that you are a student nurse/midwife because t
transition has been so quick.

This is a crucial time for you to maintain and develop your knowledge and skills and yc
positive attitude to your profession. It is so easy to fit into the team and get lost within
Now you need to remember that you are accountable for your practice so ensure that y
get the right support!

It is common in healthcare practice to have a clinical and managerial supervision structu
so check out their policies and how they provide supervision. Clinical supervision
usually monthly, often supervisee led, so use this opportunity to set the agenda, and u
it as a vehicle to reflect on your practice. You may be able to choose your supervi:
so find someone suitable for you. You might also want to attend any internal traini
workshops that will help you to get the most out of the supervision. Managerial supervisi
on the other hand, is predominantly supervisor led and looks at your performance a
practitioner and employee. Ensure that you are allocated a supervisor – this can be valua
to help you adjust to your new role and will help you to develop your knowledge a
skills.

As a novice professional you will commence the preceptorship programme which usua
runs for one year. It is essential to ensure that a newly qualified registered nurse
midwife is properly supported when they first start work. The purpose of preceptorsh
is to provide a smooth transition from the academic demands of your programme to t
practical demands of work as a registered nurse or midwife.

It is also a good idea to make contact with other professionals who work with clients
your area. Other members of the multiprofessional team can be an important source
information and knowledge for you and will help you to develop important networks a
working relationships

You are most likely to have access to an occupational health department and they are r
only used when you need vaccination boosters! The department can help with perso

problems, stress management, counselling, help you manage physical problems in your workplace and assist returning back to work after sickness.

Maintaining Your Portfolio and Developing Your Career

At the start of your professional career you need to maintain a portfolio. A portfolio is a collection of documentary evidence which is a record of your professional development. You probably had one as a student where you recorded evidence of your learning needs during the programme.

Your professional portfolio can be used to assist you in reflecting on your own professional practice as well as demonstrating to others the quality of the work you have been doing. The portfolio includes documents and materials which collectively suggest the scope and quality of your career performance.

Your portfolio is important to your development and it is up to you how you compile it. The best advice is to do it as you go along. Documenting clinical and managerial supervision sessions, your updated curriculum vitae and application form, development plans linked from appraisals, certificates of courses attended can all go in there.

Your portfolio should be used as a necessary structure for self-reflection. The process of compiling a portfolio enables you to identify both strengths and areas for development in your work performance. It allows you to plan the action you are going to take to respond to challenges and to maintain or improve your work performance. It may be used to support an application for promotion in the future or when you apply for another post.

It is worth noting that portfolios are used universally in all career pathways but they are increasingly being demanded in the nursing profession to ensure continued registration as a practitioner (NMC 2004). The portfolio helps to maintain your knowledge and competencies through lifelong learning (NMC 2002). The NMC encourages this and on renewal of registration you might be asked to demonstrate evidence of undertaking minimum hours in clinical practice and continuing professional development (NMC 2005).

Lastly, as your portfolio develops over time you will be able to identify interests in your field and this will shape your career. So look after it and use it to its full potential as it will be the basis of your practice. Good luck and enjoy your nursing or midwifery career!

Tips

- Do your homework! Ensure that the post is the right one for you
- Spend some time thinking about likely questions you will be asked at the interview
- Research issues that you suspect may be asked about at the interview
- Complete your application form thoroughly and legibly
- Ask questions at the interview, especially career development opportunities
- Think about your accountability and ensure that you get the right support to help succeed in the post
- Maintain your professional portfolio.

References

Nursing and Midwifery Council (NMC) (2002) *Supporting Nurses and Midwives Thro* *Lifelong Learning.* London, NMC.

Nursing and Midwifery Council (NMC) (2004) *Code of Professional Conduct: Standard* *Conduct, Performance and Ethics.* London, NMC.

Nursing and Midwifery Council (NMC) (2005) *The PREP Handbook.* London, NMC.

Further Reading

Hinchliff, S. Norman, S. and Schober, J. (eds) (2003) *Nursing Practice and Health Care.* edn. London, Arnold.

Department of Health (2006) *Agenda for Change* [online]. DoH, London. Avail from: http://www.dh.gov.uk/PolicyAndGuidance/HumanResources Training/ModernisingPay/AgendaForChange/fs/en

NHS Employers. (2006) *Improving Working Lives* [online]. The NHS Confederation (Emp ers) Company Ltd, London. Available from: http://www.nhsemployers.o excellence/excellence-342.cfm

NHS Plus (2006) *All about Occupation Health* [online]. DoH, London. Available f http://www.nhsplus.nhs.uk/allaboutoh/allaboutoh.asp

Nursing and Midwifery Council (2006) *Clinical Supervision* [online]. NMC, London. Avai from: http://www.nmc-uk.org/aFrameDisplay.aspx?DocumentID=1558

Nursing and Midwifery Council (2006) *Personal Professional Profiles* [online]. NMC, London. Available from: `http://www.nmc-uk.org/aFrameDisplay.aspx?DocumentID=1583`

Nursing and Midwifery Council (2006) *Preceptorship* [online]. NMC, London. Available from: http://www.nmc-uk.org/aFrameDisplay.aspx?DocumentID=1585

Chapter 23

Succeeding in Your Nursing and Midwifery Career

by Steve Trenoweth and Eddie Meyler

Choose a job you love, and you will never have to work a day in your life.
Confucius 551 BC – 478 BC

This book will have taken you on a journey from thinking and deciding about the in
application for a nursing/midwifery programme to consideration of your future ca
plans. We have offered you some guidance, advice and information on a range of iss
from the application process, to getting the best out of the interview, developing
skills of critical appraisal of the literature, getting the most out of IT, to effectively work
with your personal tutor, how to get the best out of the students' union, the student
disability, chronic health or learning needs and so forth.

The content of the chapters focused on how to succeed in nursing/midwifery educa
and included useful tips, websites and further reading. We believe the book will serve
companion to enable you to meet the requirements for registration with the Nursing
Midwifery Council (NMC) as a nurse or midwife and achieve an academic qualificatio
degree or diploma level.

We acknowledged the many challenges that you could face at both a personal
intellectual level – from the experiences of working in practice, surviving the clinical are
coping with the demands of personal and academic life. We acknowledged that you
change in a positive way as a result of your experiences in undertaking nursing/midw
education. However, we are cognizant of the stress of studying at university and
demands of learning in practice and trust that you have found the advice in the b
thought provoking and helpful.

 # *Career Pathways*

Now to briefly consider your future career opportunities. There will be opportunities for
to develop in aspects of practice related to midwifery or your chosen branch of nurs
You may find the NHS Careers website (www.nhscareers.nhs.uk/home.htm
useful resource to help you consider the various and diverse opportunities open to
It is not uncommon for nurses/midwives to view their profession as an opportunit
travel and to gain experience of health care in other parts of the world. Within the Ur
Kingdom there are career opportunities within the National Health Service (NHS),
newly qualified nurses and midwives are increasingly opting to seek employment in

independent or private sector. Today, there are a number of career pathways that you may wish to consider, such as Clinical Specialism, Management, Education, Research and Nurse Consultancy.

Succeeding in Your Nursing and Midwifery Career

Wherever you wish to take your career, and whichever pathway you choose to take, there are a number of issues you will need to consider. Completing your nursing and midwifery education is the beginning of a much longer journey – that of continually improving and developing your knowledge and skills, and becoming a lifelong learner.

You may already have some ideas about how you might want your career to progress and develop. Wherever you see yourself going, you need to be mindful of the fact that health care is continually evolving not only in terms of service provision but also in our knowledge and understanding of health and illness.

To survive in your career, you will need to ensure that you remain up to date and, as a qualified practitioner, you must be mindful of your accountability to the public. It is a professional imperative that your practice is based on sound and contemporary evidence. This will mean that you will need to take advantage of post-registration education and training opportunities that are available to you – from workshops, seminars, interprofessional learning opportunities to more formal programmes leading to higher academic awards.

However, you will need to be actively engaged in this process and committed to taking responsibility for your own ongoing personal and professional development. This process, as with all education, is facilitated by your self-awareness of, and honesty regarding, your own learning. Lifelong learning, however, is a much wider issue than attending courses or training events. Of equal value is the time you spend in personal research to find answers to questions posed by your experience in clinical practice and in your pursuit of excellence in patient care.

A Modern Career

The nursing and midwifery professions are currently undergoing major change to reflect the diverse and complex needs and wants of society. More than ever, there is a greater level of expectation from a more informed public who wish to engage in partnershi▪ healthcare delivery. This places a greater onus on future nurses and midwives to en▪ that they are capable of supporting such developments. The *Modernising Nursing Car▪* document (Department of Health 2006, p.17) outlines how nurses, for example, will lea▪ the delivery of care that patients really want. Key priority areas will be:

- Develop a competent and flexible nursing workforce
- Update career pathways and career choices
- Prepare nurses to lead in a changed healthcare system
- Modernize the image of nursing and nursing careers.

Completing your nursing and midwifery education is not really the end of the beginn▪ but the start of an exciting journey to influence healthcare practice. However, the pos▪ impact that you can make on people's lives is where real success lies. As Martin Luther ▪ Jr. (1929–68) once said:

> All labour that uplifts humanity has dignity and importance and should be undertaken wi▪ painstaking excellence.

 # *Reference*

Department of Health (2006) *Modernising Nursing Careers: Setting the Direction.* Avai▪ at: www.dh.gov.uk/assetRoot/04/13/87/57/04138757.pdf

Appendix 1

The NMC Code of Professional Conduct: Standards for Conduct, Performance and Ethics (2004)

As a registered nurse, midwife or specialist community public health nurse, you personally accountable for your practice. In caring for patients and clients, you must:

- respect the patient or client as an individual
- obtain consent before you give any treatment or care
- protect confidential information
- co-operate with others in the team
- maintain your professional knowledge and competence
- be trustworthy
- act to identify and minimise risk to patients and clients.

These are the shared values of all the United Kingdom health care regulatory bodies.

1 Introduction

1.1 The purpose of The NMC code of professional conduct: standards for cond performance and ethics is to:

- inform the professions of the standard of professional conduct required of them in exercise of their professional accountability and practice
- inform the public, other professions and employers of the standard of professio conduct that they can expect of a registered practitioner.

1.2 As a registered nurse, midwife or specialist community public health nurse, you m

- protect and support the health of individual patients and clients
- protect and support the health of the wider community
- act in such a way that justifies the trust and confidence the public have in you
- uphold and enhance the good reputation of the professions.

1.3 You are personally accountable for your practice. This means that you are answer for your actions and omissions, regardless of advice or directions from another professio

1.4 You have a duty of care to your patients and clients, who are entitled to receive and competent care.

1.5 You must adhere to the laws of the country in which you are practising.

2 As a registered nurse, midwife or specialist community public health nurse, you must respect the patient or client as an individual

2.1 You must recognise and respect the role of patients and clients as partners in their care and the contribution they can make to it. This involves identifying their preferences regarding care and respecting these within the limits of professional practice, existing legislation, resources and the goals of the therapeutic relationship.

2.2 You are personally accountable for ensuring that you promote and protect the interests and dignity of patients and clients, irrespective of gender, age, race, ability, sexuality, economic status, lifestyle, culture and religious or political beliefs.

2.3 You must, at all times, maintain appropriate professional boundaries in the relationships you have with patients and clients. You must ensure that all aspects of the relationship focus exclusively upon the needs of the patient or client.

2.4 You must promote the interests of patients and clients. This includes helping individuals and groups gain access to health and social care, information and support relevant to their needs.

2.5 You must report to a relevant person or authority, at the earliest possible time, any conscientious objection that may be relevant to your professional practice. You must continue to provide care to the best of your ability until alternative arrangements are implemented.

3 As a registered nurse, midwife or specialist community public health nurse, you must obtain consent before you give any treatment or care

3.1 All patients and clients have a right to receive information about their condition. You must be sensitive to their needs and respect the wishes of those who refuse or are unable to receive information about their condition. Information should be accurate, truthful and presented in such a way as to make it easily understood. You may need to seek legal or professional advice or guidance from your employer, in relation to the giving or withholding of consent.

3.2 You must respect patients' and clients' autonomy – their right to decide whether or not to undergo any health care intervention – even where a refusal may result in harm or death to themselves or a foetus, unless a court of law orders to the contrary. This right

is protected in law, although in circumstances where the health of the foetus would
severely compromised by any refusal to give consent, it would be appropriate to disc
this matter fully within the team and with a supervisor of midwives, and possibly to se
external advice and guidance (see clause 4).

3.3 When obtaining valid consent, you must be sure that it is:

- given by a legally competent person
- given voluntarily
- informed.

3.4 You should presume that every patient and client is legally competent unless otherv
assessed by a suitably qualified practitioner. A patient or client who is legally compet
can understand and retain treatment information and can use it to make an inforn
choice.

3.5 Those who are legally competent may give consent in writing, orally or by co-operati
They may also refuse consent. You must ensure that all your discussions and associa
decisions relating to obtaining consent are documented in the patient's or client's hea
care records.

3.6 When patients or clients are no longer legally competent and have lost the capa
to consent to or refuse treatment and care, you should try to find out whether they h
previously indicated preferences in an advance statement. You must respect any refusa
treatment or care given when they were legally competent, provided that the decisio
clearly applicable to the present circumstances and that there is no reason to believe t
they have changed their minds. When such a statement is not available, the patients
clients' wishes, if known, should be taken into account. If these wishes are not known,
criteria for treatment must be that it is in their best interests.

3.7 The principles of obtaining consent apply equally to those people who have a me
illness. Whilst you should be involved in their assessment, it will also be necessary
involve relevant people close to them; this may include a psychiatrist. When patients
clients are detained under statutory powers (mental health acts), you must ensure that
know the circumstances and safeguards needed for providing treatment and care with
consent.

3.8 In emergencies where treatment is necessary to preserve life, you may provide care without consent, if a patient or client is unable to give it, provided you can demonstrate that you are acting in their best interests.

3.9 No-one has the right to give consent on behalf of another competent adult. In relation to obtaining consent for a child, the involvement of those with parental responsibility in the consent procedure is usually necessary, but will depend on the age and understanding of the child. If the child is under the age of 16 in England and Wales, 12 in Scotland and 17 in Northern Ireland, you must be aware of legislation and local protocols relating to consent.

3.10 Usually the individual performing a procedure should be the person to obtain the patient's or client's consent. In certain circumstances, you may seek consent on behalf of colleagues if you have been specially trained for that specific area of practice.

3.11 You must ensure that the use of complementary or alternative therapies is safe and in the interests of patients and clients. This must be discussed with the team as part of the therapeutic process and the patient or client must consent to their use.

4 As a registered nurse, midwife or specialist community public health nurse, you must co-operate with others in the team

4.1 The team includes the patient or client, the patient's or client's family, informal carers and health and social care professionals in the National Health Service, independent and voluntary sectors.

4.2 You are expected to work co-operatively within teams and to respect the skills, expertise and contributions of your colleagues. You must treat them fairly and without discrimination.

4.3 You must communicate effectively and share your knowledge, skill and expertise with other members of the team as required for the benefit of patients and clients.

4.4 Health care records are a tool of communication within the team. You must ensure that the health care record for the patient or client is an accurate account of treatment, care planning and delivery. It should be consecutive, written with the involvement of the patient or client wherever practicable and completed as soon as possible after an event has occurred. It should provide clear evidence of the care planned, the decisions made, the care delivered and the information shared.

4.5 When working as a member of a team, you remain accountable for your professic conduct, any care you provide and any omission on your part.

4.6 You may be expected to delegate care delivery to others who are not registe nurses or midwives. Such delegation must not compromise existing care but must directed to meeting the needs and serving the interests of patients and clients. remain accountable for the appropriateness of the delegation, for ensuring that person who does the work is able to do it and that adequate supervision or suppo provided.

4.7 You have a duty to co-operate with internal and external investigations.

5 As a registered nurse, midwife or specialist community public health nurse, must protect confidential information

5.1 You must treat information about patients and clients as confidential and use it c for the purposes for which it was given. As it is impractical to obtain consent every t you need to share information with others, you should ensure that patients and clie understand that some information may be made available to other members of the te involved in the delivery of care. You must guard against breaches of confidentiality protecting information from improper disclosure at all times.

5.2 You should seek patients' and clients' wishes regarding the sharing of informa with their family and others. When a patient or client is considered incapable of gi permission, you should consult relevant colleagues.

5.3 If you are required to disclose information outside the team that will have pers consequences for patients or clients, you must obtain their consent. If the patient or c withholds consent, or if consent cannot be obtained for whatever reason, disclosures be made only where:

• they can be justified in the public interest (usually where disclosure is essential to pro the patient or client or someone else from the risk of significant harm)
• they are required by law or by order of a court.

5.4 Where there is an issue of child protection, you must act at all times in accordance national and local policies.

6 As a registered nurse, midwife or specialist community public health nurse, you must maintain your professional knowledge and competence

6.1 You must keep your knowledge and skills up-to-date throughout your working life. In particular, you should take part regularly in learning activities that develop your competence and performance.

6.2 To practise competently, you must possess the knowledge, skills and abilities required for lawful, safe and effective practice without direct supervision. You must acknowledge the limits of your professional competence and only undertake practice and accept responsibilities for those activities in which you are competent.

6.3 If an aspect of practice is beyond your level of competence or outside your area of registration, you must obtain help and supervision from a competent practitioner until you and your employer consider that you have acquired the requisite knowledge and skill.

6.4 You have a duty to facilitate students of nursing, midwifery and specialist community public health nursing and others to develop their competence.

6.5 You have a responsibility to deliver care based on current evidence, best practice and, where applicable, validated research when it is available.

7 As a registered nurse, midwife or specialist community public health nurse, you must be trustworthy

7.1 You must behave in a way that upholds the reputation of the professions. Behaviour that compromises this reputation may call your registration into question even if is not directly connected to your professional practice.

7.2 You must ensure that your registration status is not used in the promotion of commercial products or services, declare any financial or other interests in relevant organisations providing such goods or services and ensure that your professional judgement is not influenced by any commercial considerations.

7.3 When providing advice regarding any product or service relating to your professional role or area of practice, you must be aware of the risk that, on account of your professional title or qualification, you could be perceived by the patient or client as endorsing the product.

7.4 You should fully explain the advantages and disadvantages of alternative products that the patient or client can make an informed choice. Where you recommend a spec product, you must ensure that your advice is based on evidence and is not for your o commercial gain.

7.5 You must refuse any gift, favour or hospitality that might be interpreted, now or in future, as an attempt to obtain preferential consideration.

7.6 You must neither ask for nor accept loans from patients, clients or their relatives a friends.

8 As a registered nurse, midwife or specialist community public health nurse, y must act to identify and minimise the risk to patients and clients

8.1 You must work with other members of the team to promote health care environme that are conducive to safe, therapeutic and ethical practice.

8.2 You must act quickly to protect patients and clients from risk if you have good rea to believe that you or a colleague, from your own or another profession, may not be fi practise for reasons of conduct, health or competence. You should be aware of the te of legislation that offer protection for people who raise concerns about health and sa issues.

8.3 Where you cannot remedy circumstances in the environment of care that cc jeopardise standards of practice, you must report them to a senior person with suffic authority to manage them and also, in the case of midwifery, to the supervisor of midwi This must be supported by a written record.

8.4 When working as a manager, you have a duty toward patients and clients, colleag the wider community and the organisation in which you and your colleagues work. W facing professional dilemmas, your first consideration in all activities must be the inter and safety of patients and clients.

8.5 In an emergency, in or outside the work setting, you have a professional duty to pro care. The care provided would be judged against what could reasonably be expe from someone with your knowledge, skills and abilities when placed in those partic circumstances.

9 Indemnity insurance

9.1 The NMC recommends that a registered nurse, midwife or specialist community public health nurse, in advising, treating and caring for patients/clients, has professional indemnity insurance. This is in the interests of clients, patients and registrants in the event of claims of professional negligence.

9.2 Some employers accept vicarious liability for the negligent acts and/or omissions of their employees. Such cover does not normally extend to activities undertaken outside the registrant's employment.

9.3 Independent practice would not normally be covered by vicarious liability, while agency work may not. It is the individual registrant's responsibility to establish their insurance status and take appropriate action. In situations where employers do not accept vicarious liability, the NMC recommends that registrants obtain adequate professional indemnity insurance. If unable to secure professional indemnity insurance, a registrant will need to demonstrate that all their clients/patients are fully informed of this fact and the implications this might have in the event of a claim for professional negligence.

Glossary

Accountable Responsible for something or to someone.

Care To provide help or comfort.

Competent Possessing the skills and abilities required for lawful, safe and effective professional practice without direct supervision.

Patient and client Any individual or group using a health service.

Reasonable The case of Bolam v Friern Hospital Management Committee (1957) produced the following definition of what is reasonable. "The test is the standard of the ordinary skilled man exercising and professing to have that special skill. A man need not possess the highest expert skill at the risk of being found negligent. . . it is sufficient if he exercises the skill of an ordinary man exercising that particular art." This definition is supported and clarified by the case of Bolitho v City and Hackney Health Authority (1993).

Summary

As a registered nurse, midwife or specialist community public health nurse, you mu

- respect the patient or client as an individual
- obtain consent before you give any treatment or care
- co-operate with others in the team
- protect confidential information
- maintain your professional knowledge and competence
- be trustworthy
- act to identify and minimise the risk to patients and clients

Reproduced with permission of the Nursing and Midwifery Council

Appendix 2

**An NMC Guide For Students
Of Nursing And Midwifery
Updated 2005**

Welcome to your programme of nursing or midwifery education. Choosing to becom
nurse of midwife is a big step, but it means that you are on the way to becoming on
the most important people in society. Patients and the public truly value the work you
be doing when you qualify.

Once you have successfully completed your programme of education, you will need
register with the Nursing and Midwifery Council (NMC) before you can practise as a nu
or midwife.

This leaflet sets out some basic information about the NMC and some guidance for
clinical experience you will undertake during your studies. It is based upon extensive c
sultation with individual pre-registration students of nursing and midwifery, organisati
representing students and lecturers in higher education.

The leaflet should be read in conjunction with advice provided by your higher educat
institution.

 ## *What Does the NMC do?*

The NMC is the regulatory body for nursing and midwifery. Our purpose is to estab
and improve standards of nursing and midwifery care in order to protect the public. Th
standards are set out in The NMC code of professional conduct: standards for cond
performance and ethics, which the NMC will send to you when you first register. We u
you to get hold of a copy now. You should be able to obtain it through your universit
not, it's on our web site at www.nmc-uk.org

You may not be aware that the standards set by the NMC already apply to you. The le
of entry to the programme of education that you are undertaking and the content, t
and length of your programme are all part of these standards. The NMC has other
responsibilities which are to:

- maintain a register of qualified nurses and midwives
- set standards for nursing and midwifery education, performance, ethics and conduct
- provide advice and guidance on professional standards
- consider allegations of unfitness to practise due to misconduct, ill health or lack
  competence.

Registration and Professional Accountability

When you successfully complete your course, your higher education institution will notify the NMC that you have met the required standards and that you are eligible for entry on the register. Your course director will also complete a declaration of good health and good character on your behalf. When we have received this information and you have paid your registration fee, your name will be entered on the NMC register and you will be eligible to practise as a registered practitioner. This should take a matter of days. Registration is not simply an administrative process. The NMC's register is an instrument of public protection and anyone can check the registered status of a nurse or midwife.

Registering with the NMC demonstrates that you have met the standards expected of registered nurses and midwives. It also demonstrates that you are professionally accountable at all times for your acts and omissions.

Professional accountability involves weighing up the interests of patients and clients, using your professional judgement and skills to make a decision and enabling you to account for the decision you make. On rare occasions, nurses and midwives fall short of the professional standards expected of them. The NMC investigates in the public interest any complaints made about the professional conduct or fitness to practise of registered nurses and midwives.

Throughout your career, you will need to keep up to date with developments in your area of practice. Your continuing professional development is an integral part of your professional accountability. In order to continue to practise, you will need to meet the NMC's standards for post-registration education and practice (PREP). Detailed information about PREP is available in The PREP Handbook, which you can download from the NMC web site, or obtain free of charge from our Publications Department. You will also need to complete a notification of practice form when you renew your registration every three years and pay your annual retention fee. Practising midwives also need to complete a notification of intention to practise form annually.

Guidance on clinical experience for students

During your studentship, you will come into close contact with patients or clients. This may be through observing care being given, through helping in providing care and, later,

through full participation in providing care. At all times, you should work only within yc
level of understanding and competence, and always under the appropriate supervision
a registered nurse or midwife, or a health professional with a registered nurse or midwe
providing mentorship.

The section below provides some guidance on working with patients or clients duri
your studies. The principles underpinning this guidance reflect the standards that will
expected of you when you become a registered practitioner.

Your Accountability

As a pre-registration student, you are not professionally accountable in the way that y
will be after you come to register with the NMC. This means that you cannot be called
account for your actions and omissions by the NMC. So far as the NMC is concerned, it is t
registered practitioners with whom you are working who are professionally responsible
the consequences of your actions and omissions. This is why you must always work und
direct supervision. This does not mean, however, that you can never be called to accou
by your university or by the law for the consequences of your actions or omissions a
pre-registration student.

The Wishes of Patients

You must respect the wishes of patients and clients at all times. They have the right
refuse to allow you, as a student, to participate in caring for them and you should make t
right clear to them when they are first given information about the care they will rece
from you. You should leave if they ask you to do so. Their rights, as patients or clier
supersede at all times your rights to knowledge and experience.

Identifying Yourself

You should introduce yourself accurately at all times when speaking to patients or clie
either directly or by telephone. In doing so, you should make it quite clear that you
a pre-registration student and not a registered practitioner. In fact, it is a criminal offer
for anyone to represent him or herself falsely and deliberately as a registered nurse
midwife.

Accepting Appropriate Responsibility

There may be times when you are in a position where you may not be directly accompanied by your mentor, supervisor or another registered colleague, such as emergency situations. As your skills, experience and confidence develop, you will become increasingly able to deal with these situations. However, as a student, do not participate in any procedure for which you have not been fully prepared or in which you are not adequately supervised. If such a situation arises, discuss the matter as quickly as possible with your mentor or personal tutor.

Patient Confidentiality

Patients have the right to know that any private and personal information that is given in confidence will be used only for the purposes for which it was originally provided and that it will not be used for any other reason.

If you want to refer in a written assignment to some real-life situation in which you have been involved, do not provide any information that could identify a particular patient or client. Obtain access to patient records only when absolutely necessary for the care being provided. Use of these records must be closely supervised by a registered practitioner and you must follow the local policy on the handling and storage of records. Any written entry you make in a patient's or clients records must be counter-signed by a registered practitioner. You can find more advice about confidentiality in The NMC code of professional conduct: standards for conduct, performance and ethics. You should also refer to our Guidelines for records and record keeping.

Handling Complaints

You will need to be aware of the local procedures for dealing with complaints by patients, clients, or their families, about the treatment or care they are receiving. If patients indicate to you that they are unhappy about their treatment or care, you should report the matter immediately to the person who is supervising your clinical experience or to another appropriate person.

What If I See Something I Think is Wrong?

As a student, you will experience a range of different settings in your practice education placements. You will be well placed to question why something is or is not being done.

In some cases, you may see a registered nurse or midwife doing something you fee inappropriate. Although difficult, you shouldn't ignore the situation. Ask the person someone else about it.

In some cases, you may be observing what could amount to misconduct. Whether or this is the case, challenging experienced practitioners' ways of doing things should encouraged. This will show you are observing and thinking, and may help a practitio improve their own practice.

We hope that you will find these notes helpful during your programme and in und standing the important responsibilities you will later undertake as a registered nurse midwife.

If you need to discuss any of these issues with us, please contact our professional adv service on 020 7333 6541/6550/6553, by e-mail at advice@nmc-uk.org or by fax on 7333 6538.

If you would like to find out more about the work of the NMC, our website at www.nm uk.org includes copies of all NMC publications, position statements issued by professional advice service, and further useful information and contacts for student nursing and midwifery.

Good luck in your programme of preparation for registration and in your future career.

Published by the former United Kingdom Central Council for Nursing, Midwifery and Healt Visiting in July 1998

Reprinted by the Nursing and Midwifery Council in April 2002

Updated by the Nursing and Midwifery Council in December 2005

Reproduced with Permission of the Nursing and Midwifery Council

Appendix 3

A Quick Guide to Harvard Referencing

Please note this is not an exhaustive list and you are advised to refer to any guidance giv
by your university in the first instance.

Acknowledging Authors in Your Text

- CITATIONS – SINGLE AUTHOR

> There are many different forms of knowledge that nurses appear to use to underpin
> their practice (Carper 1978).

Or:

> According to Carper (1978), there are many different forms of knowledge that nurses
> appear to use to underpin their practice.

- CITATIONS – MULTIPLE AUTHORS
  When there are two authors, it is usual to cite both:

> Homoeostasis is an important concept in providing holistic mental health nursing
> care (Rinomhota and Marshall 2000).

But when there are two or more authors, it is usual to cite the first author followed
'et al' (meaning 'and others')

> The perception of our 'self' can be seen as being partly determined by our cultural
> frame of reference (Walker et al 2004).

- CITATIONS BY SAME AUTHOR IN SAME YEAR

> One of the most important roles of the Nursing and Midwifery Council (NMC) is to
> deal with allegations relating to a nurse or midwife's fitness to practise (NMC 2004a;
> NMC 2004b).

Here, you are citing two documents published by the Nursing and Midwifery Council in the same year. The convention is use sequential letters of the alphabet. In your reference list you will cite the following:

> NMC (2004a) *Complaints about unfitness to practise: A guide for members of the public.* London, NMC.
> NMC (2004b) *Reporting unfitness to practise: for employers managers.* London, NMC.

If you refer to the *Complaints about unfitness to practise: A guide for members of the public* elsewhere in your essay you will continue to reference this as NMC (2004a).

- SECONDARY REFERENCES

> For Seligman (1975 cited in Walker et al 2004), depression could arise if one felt that one's actions could not influence an outcome of an event.

Note: In your reference list you list Walker et al (2004) only.

- AUTHORED WEBSITES

Here you will cite the author and the date (if known) as above. If the date is not known you will use 'n.d.' e.g. Smith (n.d.).

- NON-AUTHORED WEBSITES

> Good infection control nursing will help to stop the spread of *Clostridium difficile* disease (DoH 2006)

See below for guidance on how to reference websites.

- DIRECT QUOTATIONS

> The family or caregiver can provide a timeline history of the illness and precipitants to the current event (Jones 2005, 21) or (Jones 2005, p. 21)

If the quote continues over two pages or more it is usual to use the abbreviation 'pp' (simply meaning 'pages').

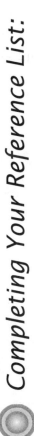

Completing Your Reference List:

All references must be listed alphabetically in a consistent style (e.g. using the same font, spacing and punctuation)

1.   AN AUTHORED BOOK

Campbell, J. (2003) *Campbell's Physiology Notes for Nurses*. London, Whurr.

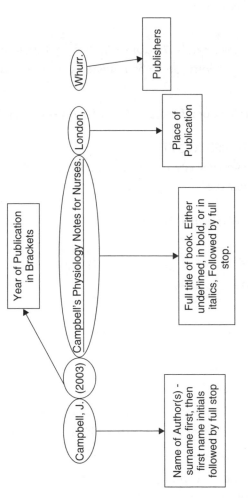

2. AN EDITED BOOK

Jones, B.(2005) A carer's perspective of care planning. In: Tummey, R. (ed). *Planning Care in Mental Health Nursing*. Basingstoke, Palgrave.

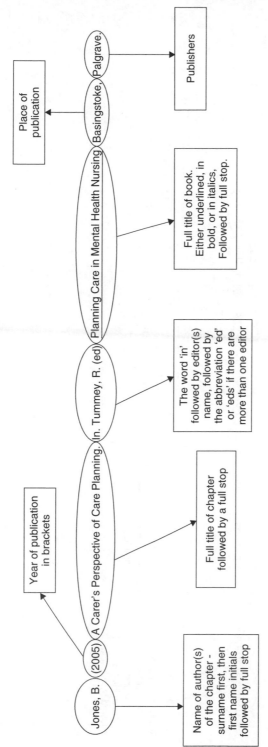

Year of publication in brackets

Name of author(s) of the chapter - surname first, then first name initials followed by full stop

Full title of chapter followed by a full stop

The word 'in' followed by editor(s) name, followed by the abbreviation 'ed' or 'eds' if there are more than one editor

Full title of book. Either underlined, in bold, or in italics. Followed by full stop.

Place of publication

Publishers

3.   A JOURNAL ARTICLE

Carper, B. (1978) Fundamental patterns of knowing in nursing. Advances in Nursing Science. **1**(1), 13 – 23.

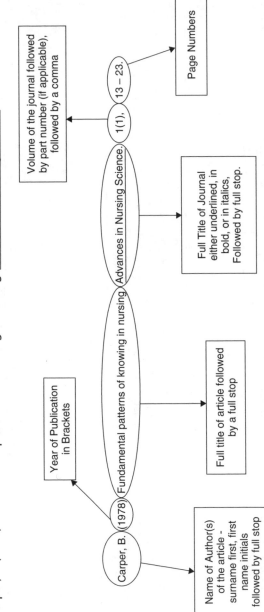

4. ELECTRONIC SOURCES

Department of Health (DoH) (2006) *A Simple Guide To Clostridium Difficile.*

Available from: www.dh.gov.uk/PolicyAndGuidance/HealthAndSocialCareTopics/HealthcareAcquiredInfection/fs/en [Accessed 7 November 2006]

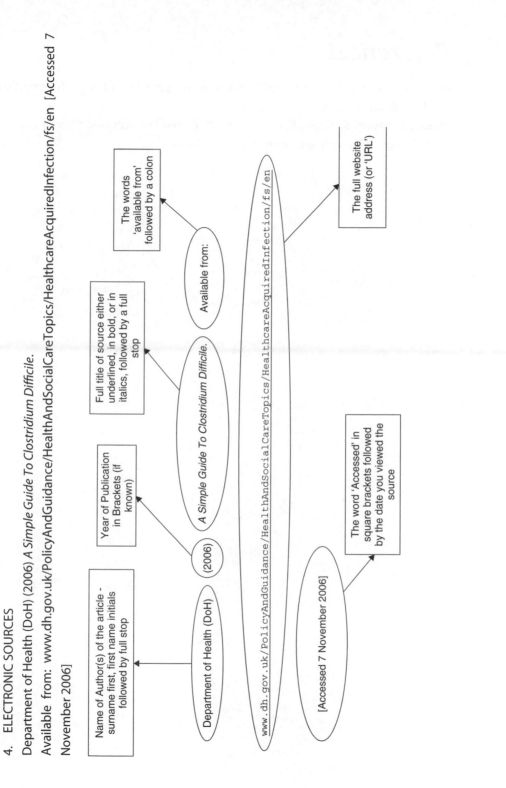

References

Rinomhota, A. and Marshall, P. (2000) *Biological Aspects of Mental Health Nursing*. Edinbur Churchill Livingstone.

Walker, J., Payne, S., Smith, P. and Jarrett, N. (2004) *Psychology for Nurses and the Ca Professions*. Maidenhead, Open University Press.

List of Contributors

Eddie Meyler MSc, BA (Hons), RMN, RGN, RNT Cert Ed.   Director of Studies, Thames Valley University. Eddie has, since 1994, managed and developed the mental health branch of the pre-registration nursing programme at Thames Valley University. Eddie has a keen interest in supporting students classed as being 'non-standard entrants' undertaking a career in nursing. Currently, as Director of Studies, Eddie has responsibly for promoting the students' learning experience across all branches of nursing. This book is a culmination of his appreciation of a need for a resource to help students achieve success in their chosen health care career

Steve Trenoweth MSc, BSc (Hons) Psychology, PGDipEA, RMN, ILTM   Senior Lecturer, Thames Valley University. Steve has been a Senior Lecturer since 2003, prior to which he was a Lecturer/Practitioner in Forensic Mental Health Services. His clinical interests include the improvement of physical health amongst mental health clients, risk assessment, psychosocial assessment and interventions and personal construct therapy/psychology. His doctoral research is the study of personal change amongst mental health nursing students as they progress through their programme.

Sue McGowan   Student Nurse, Thames Valley University. Sue finished full time education 21 years ago with a few O and A levels. She feels that she has been bitten by the education bug and would like to study further once qualified. She is particularly interested in older adult nursing and at some stage would like to specialize in dementia care. She has plans to participate in research in this field.

Denise Burley MSc, SRN, SCM, HV Cert., Dip N Ed (Lond)   Director of Studies, Thames Valley University. Denise is responsible for Post Qualifying courses at Thames Valley University. She was previously a Pathway Leader for the BSc (Hons) Health Promotion and Public Health as well as a module leader for the pre-registration module entitled 'Primary Care and Public Health'. She has been closely involved with two NHS Direct sites

and developed a module for nurses working in telephone triage, which has been furt
developed to support nurses working in other situations such as GP Surgeries. She is
a member of the editorial board of two professional journals.

David Stroud MA, BSc (Hons), RMN, RGN, RNT   Senior Lecturer, Thames Valley U
versity. David has been an independent lecturer and therapist since 1994, working b
in the NHS and privately, with a special interest in group work. He is well-known for
pioneering work in the community, which includes introducing therapy groups such
stress management, anger management and assertiveness training. He finds it natura
transfer the skills of therapy to his teaching, which is greatly appreciated by the stude
His work has included leading tutorial and supervision groups at Thames Valley Univer
Although his varied qualifications and experience have allowed him to teach on b
common foundation and mental health branch courses, his main teaching interests
centred around communication skills and reflection. He is also a qualified hypnothera
and works in both English and Spanish.

Pauline McInnes BA in Psychology and Education, Certificate in Higher Educat
and Disability Services   Disability Coordinator, Thames Valley University. Pauline
worked in the fields of Disability and Education since 1998 and for the past three ye
has been the Disability Coordinator at Thames Valley University. Over the past n
years, Pauline has worked with students with disabilities across the education sector fn
primary school aged children to adults in Further and Higher Education. Her roles h
been varied, including student casework, staff development, strategic action plann
and managing a service for disabled students. The chapter in this book is Pauline's
published work.

Ian Chisholm-Bunting BSc Biol Sci, BSC (Hons) Nursing, RGN, PDDipE, RNT   Se
Lecturer, Thames Valley University. Ian has been nursing for 19 years. His areas of inte
are organizational behaviour, management and leadership in the NHS, critical car
the adult in the hospital setting, and diabetes. Ian teaches at both undergraduate
post-graduate level and finds his students a continuing source of inspiration.

Kris Ramgoolam TD, MSc, BSc (Hons), RMN, RNMH, RN, Dip N (London), RCNT,
Ed (Nursing).   Senior Lecturer, Thames Valley University. Kris's current role is tha
Common Foundation Programme Leader to all Mental Health students. He teache
aspects of nursing, theory and practice to first year students and supports them du
clinical placement. His clinical area of interest is the cognitive processing and 'mal
meaning' of life traumatic events and its long-term beneficial effects on health.

Anthony Meyler   Anthony works as both a teacher and an IT consultant. He has built up a business of providing computer, technical and network services to both small and large infrastructures. He doubles as a teacher and private tutor facilitating essential learning at Key Stages 3 and 4. At present he has the sole responsibility for providing a new Key Stage 3 ICT Curriculum. He intends to develop a delivery method that forces a shift towards interactive independent learning.

Helen Robson RGN, RMN, RM, DPSN, BSc.   Lecturer, Thames Valley University. Since first qualifying as a nurse in 1990, most of Helen's clinical experience has been within mental health nursing, both within general and forensic services. Additionally, Helen has qualifications in Adult Nursing and is a Midwife. She moved into nurse education in 2004, and is currently completing a Masters Degree in Mental Health Care.

Dr Deirdre Kelley-Patterson, BSc Psychology, MSc Organisational Psychology, PhD
Head of Centre, Centre for the Study of Policy and Practice in Health and Social Care, Thames Valley University. Deirdre is a psychology graduate with an interest in service improvement, leadership and career development. Currently, she works with NHS and Social Care workforce planners to support and develop their skills in the commissioning and development of staff to meet the current social policy requirements.

Lai Chan Koh MBA, MA in Further and Higher Education, BA, RN, RNT   Principal Lecturer, University Teaching Fellow. Lai Chan is a Principal Lecturer in the Faculty of Health and Human Sciences at Thames Valley University. She has considerable experience in teaching the acute care of the adult patients. Her main responsibilities are in the management and development of teaching and learning in the Pre-Registration Nursing Programme. She also teaches on the MA in Teaching and Learning programme with interests in assessment and formative feedback. Other responsibilities include working with clinical practitioners to provide quality practice environments for learners. A recent addition to her role as a University Teaching Fellow extends her interests into innovation in teaching, learning and assessing learners.

Pam Louison BA, DMS, MCILIP   Subject Librarian, Thames Valley University. Pam is a qualified librarian and has many years experience of working in health sciences. She is interested in supporting and developing information skills training to enable library users to acquire the knowledge and skills to find, evaluate and utilize sources of information.

Dr Julia Magill-Cuerden PhD, MA, Dip Ed, DipN, MTD, RM, RN   Principal Lecturer, Teaching Fellow. Julia is a Fellow of the Royal College of Midwives and a National Teaching

Fellow. Her experience has been in midwifery education and she has taught student: undergraduate and post-graduate education, with a particular interest in their writ and developing skills for assessments and research dissertations. She is a Supervi of Midwives in clinical practice and an editor for a professional midwifery journal. publishes regularly, mostly in midwifery. She has a keen interest in teaching research education within the health professions, and undertaking research in education and au in clinical practice.

Samantha Torres BSc (Hons), RNMH   Clinical Team Leader. Samantha has had a k interest in education since qualifying as a nurse. She is involved with developing nursing education curriculum and also supports student nurses and mentors alike wit her role as Student Liaison on the ward where she works. She is planning to develop further by preparing to be a Practice Teacher.

Simon Jones MA (Video) MSc(Research) MA (Film) PgCert (Teach) BA (Hons)   Lectu (Research) Richard Wells Research Centre, Thames Valley University. Simon graduated fr De Montfort University in 2000 with a First Class BA (Hons) in Media Studies and A: Philosophy. Since then he has been awarded an MA in Film and MA in Video Product from the London College of Music and Media, and a Post-Graduate Certificate in Teach and an MSc in Research from Thames Valley University. He currently works for the Rich Wells Research Centre as a Lecturer (Research).

Sue Vernon BA (Hons) Humanities, PGCE   Head of Learning Skills (HE). Sue has b involved in teaching and supporting students in higher and further education for c 14 years. She has been involved in curriculum development and quality issues for a w range of courses from Access to undergraduate programmes. She has developed a v range of study skills materials both for use in the classroom and online. Her main inter are plagiarism and referencing, essay writing and exam strategies.

Deann Cox BSc, RGN   Clinical Skills Centre Co-ordinator, Thames Valley University. De qualified as a general nurse in 1979, since which she has worked the majority of the t within critical care areas specifically Anaesthesia and Cardio Thoracics. During this ti Deann completed post-registration courses in Anaesthetic Nursing and Adult Inten Care Nursing, before spending six years as a joint appointment (clinical/education) at Brompton Hospital Cardiothoracic Intensive Care Unit. Deann is currently a Clinical S Centre Coordinator, introducing a simulated clinical environment.

Stella Brophy BSc (Hons) Professional Practice with Critical Care Reg. Nurse, Reg. Midwife, Dip. Nursing (London) JBCNS (ENB100), City and Guilds 730, FETC, Cert Ed. MEd.   Principal Lecturer, Thames Valley University. Stella is a midwife but in recent years has specialised in critical care. She was a Senior Sister at St. Mary's Hospital, London, where she managed a variety of clinical services. She has been Programme Leader for many health care programmes.

Karen Elcock MSc, PgDip, BSc, RN, RNT, Cert Ed (Fe)   Project Leader for Learning Community Development, Practice Education Support Unit, Thames Valley University. Karen's professional interests are in practice education, with particular focus on how students are prepared for learning in practice, mentor development and support and the development of academic support roles to practice, with her research focussing on the latter two areas. Her published work includes papers addressing the roles of Advanced Nurse Practitioners, Consultant Nurses, Lecturer Practitioners and student nurses

Index